Published

Bleck: Orthopaedic Management of Cerebral Palsy

Jowsey: Metabolic Diseases of Bone

Forthcoming Monographs in the Series

Gustilo: Management of Open Fractures and Their Complicat

Hughston, Walsh and Puddu: Patellar Subluxation and Disloc

Nelson and Nelson: Orthopaedic Infections

Pappas and Akins: The Child's Hip

Southwick and Johnson: Surgical Approaches to the Spine

COMPARTMENT SYNDROMES AND VOLKMANN'S CONTRACTURE

by

SCOTT J. MUBARAK, M.D.

Assistant Professor
Division of Orthopaedic Surgery and Rehabilitation

and

ALAN R. HARGENS, Ph.D.

Associate Professor
Division of Orthopaedic Surgery and Rehabilitation

Volume III in the Series

SAUNDERS MONOGRAPHS
IN CLINICAL ORTHOPAEDICS

Consulting Editor
CLEMENT B. SLEDGE, M.D.

1981   W. B. SAUNDERS COMPANY
Philadelphia • London • Toronto • Sydney

W. B. Saunders Company: West Washington Square
Philadelphia, PA 19105

1 St. Anne's Road
Eastbourne, East Sussex BN21 3UN, England

1 Goldthorne Avenue
Toronto, Ontario M8Z 5T9, Canada

9 Waltham Street
Artarmon, N.S.W. 2064, Australia

Library of Congress Cataloging in Publication Data

Main entry under title:

Compartment syndromes and Volkmann's contracture.

(Saunders monographs in clinical orthopaedics; v. 3)

1. Compartment syndrome.   I. Mubarak, Scott J.
II. Hargens, Alan R.   III. Akeson, Wayne H. [DNLM:
1. Anterior compartment syndrome.   2. Volkmann's
contracture. W1 SA975 v. 3 / WE 550 M941c]

RC951.C52   616.7'4   80–52774

ISBN 0–7216–6604–3

Compartment Syndromes and Volkmann's Contracture   ISBN   0-7216-6604-3

Last digit is the print number: 9   8   7   6   5   4   3   2   1

Dedicated to our wives
Sandy *and* Gunvør
and our children
Jason, Tor, *and* Lars.

Foreword

Volkmann's ischemia with supracondylar fractures; anterior tibial syndrome after running; compartment syndromes following fractures of the extremities; ischemic nerve loss following tibial osteotomy; circumferential burns of the extremities — what surgeon doesn't face these problems frequently?

The clinical diagnosis and value of surgical decompression in ischemic compartment syndromes are concepts that have been around for nearly 100 years. What has been missing is an awareness of the frequency of this serious complication, knowledge of its pathophysiology, and — most important — reliable, objective methods to establish the diagnosis in a timely fashion.

These goals are admirably met in this monograph by Drs. Mubarak and Hargens. Clinicians will find it indispensable for increasing their awareness of the many forms of compartmental ischemia. Surgeons will find valuable guidelines for operative intervention. Investigators will find an excellent review of the pathophysiology of this condition. Surely there is something in this book for almost everyone.

The authors state that "despite an increased awareness of the problem by physicians, compartment syndromes remain poorly understood, and frequently are poorly managed. They are overlooked by physicians because: (1) the condition has multiple etiologies; (2) the incidence is relatively infrequent; (3) they are comparatively unknown to many physicians; and (4) the findings of a compartment syndrome are frequently confused with those of other disorders." This monograph should do much to reverse this deplorable situation. It is to be hoped that it will find its way *onto* every orthopedist's book shelf and *into* our methods of managing patients, thereby preventing the devastating sequelae of unrecognized and untreated compartment syndromes.

CLEMENT B. SLEDGE, M.D.

Preface

Our studies of compartment syndromes that stimulated this book began in 1973, when a first year orthopedic resident (Scott Mubarak) began collaboration with a young physiologist (Alan Hargens) to refine the wick catheter technique for clinical use. Together with the help of our mentors Wayne Akeson, M.D., Charles Owen, M.D., and P. F. Scholander, Ph.D., these investigations were undertaken.

This book combines clinical and experimental viewpoints for in-depth coverage of compartment syndromes. Its timeliness is noteworthy since much recent research has focused on the pathophysiology, prevention, diagnosis, and treatment of compartment syndromes. In particular, clinical use of intracompartmental pressure is now an important tool by which a physician may objectively assess the course of an acute compartment syndrome. The wick catheter and slit catheter techniques are commercially available today, so that the use of intracompartmental pressure is now a valuable adjunct for evaluating possible compartment syndromes.

Important experimental and clinical findings obtained within the past five years by several investigators are included. Our examination of these new experimental findings and their clinical implications fulfills another purpose of this book: namely, to combine the ideas and efforts of basic scientists with those of clinicians to understand the abnormal tissue fluid balance related to compartment syndromes. Based on these objectives, our book is primarily addressed to orthopedic surgeons and residents, medical students, researchers interested in tissue pressure and muscle circulation, and other clinicians who need an updated, detailed, and comprehensive reference that covers the history, anatomy, diagnosis, and treatment of compartment syndromes.

We are indebted to many who have contributed to this endeavor. Much of the information provided in this book resulted from clinical and experimental research that was supported by the Veterans Administration, USPHS/NIH grants AM-18824, AM-25501, AM-00602, and GM-24901, National Aeronautics and Space Administration contract NAS 9-16039, and by the Division of Orthopedics and Rehabilitation, University of California Medical Center, San Diego. We thank Debbie Guthrie and Barbara Sverdrup for their assistance in preparing the manuscript in final form and we thank Kurt Smolen for his artistic talents that are abundantly illustrated in the following pages. We also thank Larry Garetto, Karen Evans, Sanford Zweifach, John Cologne, Richard Ord, Patricia Dedrick, Ann-Kristin Lundblad, Peggie Gorball, and Albert Crenshaw for expert technical assistance and Mary Gonsalves for her excellent histologic work. We are indebted to many past orthopedic residents (Drs. Ladd Rutherford, Donald Schmidt, Steven Garfin, Robert Smith, Robert Gould, and Yu Fon Lee) for their research input and long hours with patients. And finally we thank the University of California, San Diego and our orthopedic colleagues who have contributed so much as advisors, researchers, and co-authors: Drs. Wayne Akeson, Charles Owen, Steven Garfin, David Gershuni, and Richard Gelberman.

SCOTT J. MUBARAK, M.D.

ALAN R. HARGENS, Ph.D.

Contents

Chapter One

DEFINITION AND TERMINOLOGY

Alan R. Hargens, Ph.D.,
and Scott J. Mubarak, M.D.

A *compartment syndrome* is a condition in which high pressure within a closed fascial space (muscle compartment) reduces capillary blood perfusion below a level necessary for tissue viability. The local ischemia produced by a compartment syndrome must be relieved by decompressing the muscle compartment, in order to prevent muscle and nerve necrosis. Usually, decompression is accomplished by fasciotomy, which allows the muscle to swell out of its tight fascial enclosure. The four muscle compartments of the lower leg are involved most frequently, but compartment syndromes in the forearm, arm, shoulder, thigh, and buttock also occur (see Chapter 3). Compartment syndromes develop in skeletal muscles that are enclosed by relatively noncompliant, osseofascial boundaries. A build-up of pressure within the muscle compartment is not easily dissipated, owing to the inelastic nature of the muscle-investing fascia. If pressure remains sufficiently high for several hours, normal function of the muscle and nerves is jeopardized, and myoneural necrosis eventually will result. Permanent loss of function and limb contracture may occur. A prompt diagnosis and decompression of this condition is therefore essential in order to reinstate capillary perfusion and prevent irreversible sequelae (Fig. 1–1).

Compartment syndromes are divided into two forms, acute and chronic, with regard to etiology and reversibility. An *acute* compartment syndrome is a severe form, usually following trauma, in which intracompartmental pressure is elevated to a level and duration such that decompression is necessary to prevent necrosis and preserve limb viability (see Chapters 6 and 7). Synonyms for an acute compartment syndrome are anterior tibial syndrome, calf hypertension, compartmental syndrome, Volkmann's ischemia, impending ischemic contracture, and march gangrene. Although an acute compartment syndrome most commonly confronts orthopedic surgeons in association with extremity fractures, compartment syndromes may present to any physician or specialist in association with contusions, bleeding disorders, burns, trauma, vascular repair, exercise, drug or alcohol overdose, tight dressings, venous obstruction, and other forms of ischemia (see Chapter 5).

Intracompartmental pressure is raised through any one of a number of etiologies that, in general terms, include interstitial edema, hemorrhage, or muscle fiber

1

SECTION OF MUSCLE COMPARTMENTS

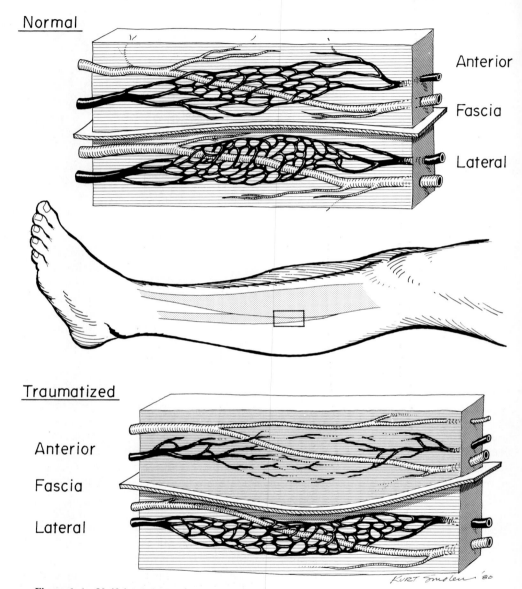

Figure 1-1 Unifying principles of a compartment syndrome. In the enlarged figure above the leg, normal microcirculation is viewed during rest in the anterior and lateral muscle compartments. These two compartments are separated by fascia. During rest, intracompartmental pressure in the anterior and lateral compartments is near zero, and blood flow in all capillaries (*network of black vessels*) and large arteries (*shaded vessels entering figure from the right*) is normal. If pressure in the anterior compartment reaches a threshold level near 30 mm Hg (*enlarged figure below leg*), capillary perfusion is inadequate to maintain tissue viability. If this high pressure in the anterior compartment is not relieved after approximately eight hours, irreversible necrosis of muscle tissue and indwelling nerves may result in the anterior compartment. It is noteworthy that distal pulses are usually present in the foot primarily because intracompartmental pressure rarely rises above central-artery diastolic pressure.

swelling within the compartment (see Chapter 4). Intracompartmental edema is produced by increased capillary permeability following burn injuries, arterial drug injection, vascular reconstruction surgery, prolonged limb compression, venous obstruction, crush injuries, and perhaps venomous snake bites. Muscle fiber swelling often follows long periods of ischemia, with subsequent abnormal intracellular ion accumulation and water uptake. Intracompartmental pressure is also elevated by compartment volume constriction (external compression, tight casts, or burn eschars).

Increased capillary hydrostatic pressure or lymphatic obstruction within the involved muscle compartment could also produce sufficient interstitial edema to initiate a syndrome. A low colloidal content in blood (for example, low plasma albumin concentrations during nephrosis) may cause a compartment syndrome by reducing transcapillary fluid resorption. Hemorrhage within the closed compartment space after major vessel laceration, hereditary hemorrhagic diathesis, fractures, or contusions may also produce a compartment syndrome. Finally, exercise combined with fascial inelasticity or muscle hypertrophy may cause an acute compartment syndrome.

A second form of compartment syndrome, the *chronic* or *exertional* compartment syndrome, occurs when exercise raises intracompartment pressure sufficiently to produce ischemia, pain, and (on rare occasions) neurologic deficit (see Chapter 14). This condition represents a mild, recurrent compartment syndrome associated with exercise in which symptoms of pain, and sometimes nerve loss, spontaneously resolve upon rest. However, if the exercise is continued despite pain and eventual neuromuscular deficit, a chronic compartment syndrome may proceed to the acute form that requires immediate decompression. A classic example of the latter is the military recruit who exercises or marches under duress beyond his own limits of pain tolerance. Synonyms for the chronic compartment syndrome include exercise ischemia, exercise myopathy, and recurrent compartment syndrome.

Whereas the term "compartment syndrome" usually refers to localized or limited myoneural ischemia, a *crush syndrome* represents the systemic manifestations of more severe muscle necrosis with multicompartment involvement (see Chapter 11). Muscle infarctions associated with crush syndromes produce myoglobinemia, extracellular fluid loss, and acidosis/hyperkalemia. In severe cases these manifestations produce renal failure, shock, and cardiac arrhythmia, respectively (Mubarak and Owen, 1975). Rhabdomyolysis is a synonym for a crush syndrome.

A *Volkmann's contracture* is a limb deformity that represents the last stage of muscle and nerve necrosis following an acute compartment syndrome. Synonyms for Volkmann's contracture include ischemic contracture, ischemic necrosis, and traumatic necrosis. This residual of a compartment syndrome was first described by von Volkmann (1875, 1881, 1882), who proposed that the syndrome was caused by tight dressings or casts applied to a traumatized extremity. Since these volume-containing enclosures restrict limb swelling, pressure rises prodigiously within tissues located inside these noncompliant containers. It is now apparent that a Volkmann's contracture may result from many circumstances other than tight dressings or casts (see Chapters 2 and 4). If the outcome of an unrelieved compartment syndrome in a limb is severe, atrophy and contracture of the involved muscles, as well as the irreversible neurologic deficit, will require reconstructive surgery (see Chapters 12 and 13).

The sequelae of an unrelieved acute compartment syndrome are devastating to the individual involved, in terms of functional disability. In its most severe form, the crush syndrome, the entity is life-threatening. Despite an increased awareness of the problem by physicians, compartment syndromes remain poorly understood, and frequently are poorly managed. They are overlooked by physicians because: (1) the condition has multiple etiologies; (2) the incidence is relatively infrequent; (3) they are comparatively unknown to many physicians; and (4) the findings of a compartment syndrome are frequently confused with those of other disorders.

Adding to the obscurity of compartment syndromes is the use of many different terms (Volkmann's ischemia, calf hypertension, anterior tibial syndrome), all of which describe the same condition of increased pressure and ischemia within a muscle compartment. Several debilitating conditions mimic the symptoms of compartment syndromes (pain, neurologic deficit, or edema). However, elevated intracompartmental pressure is absent in these conditions, and thus there is none of the intrinsic muscle and nerve ischemia that characterizes all compartment syndromes. Some of these conditions include stress fractures, arterial injury (compensated occlusion), direct nerve contusion, cellulitis, snake bites, and perhaps shin splints (Mubarak et al., 1978; Garfin et al., 1979).

The clinical findings of a compartment syndrome are rather subjective, and rely heavily on patient cooperation. Therefore, an equilibrium measurement of intracompartmental pressure offers an important adjunct to diagnostic procedures. Pressure measurements enable the physician to evaluate and monitor compartment syndromes more objectively. Ideally, with prompt diagnosis, early and effective treatment is accomplished and normal function of the limb is maintained (see Chapters 8–10).

In the past two decades important advances have been made in revealing the pathophysiology of compartment syndromes. Chronic compartment syndromes, initiated by exercise, were studied in depth by Reneman (1968) for the anterior and lateral compartments of the leg. Whitesides et al. (1971) described the histologic response of skeletal muscle to tourniquet ischemia of various durations. Matsen's classification (1975) clarified the multiplicity of injuries and diseases associated with compartment syndromes. Rorabeck and Clarke's important study of pressure and time variables in dogs (1978) helped identify threshold pressure parameters that produce compartmental injury. These studies and others, including the authors' research on compartment syndromes, are covered in subsequent chapters of this book.

REFERENCES

Garfin, S. R., Davidson, T. M., and Mubarak, S. J.: Rattlesnake bites: current concepts. Clin. Orthop. 140:50–57, 1979.

Matsen, F. A., III: Compartmental syndrome: a unified concept. Clin. Orthop. 113:8–13, 1975.

Mubarak, S. J., and Owen, C. A.: Compartment syndrome and its relation to the crush syndrome: a spectrum of disease. Clin. Orthop. 113:81–89, 1975.

Mubarak, S. J., Owen, C. A., Hargens, A. R., Garetto, L. P., and Akeson, W. H.: Acute compartment syndromes: diagnosis and treatment with the aid of the wick catheter. J. Bone Joint Surg. 60A:1091–1095, 1978.

Reneman, R. S.: The Anterior and the Lateral Compartment Syndrome of the Leg. Mouton Co., The Hague, 1968.

Rorabeck, C. H., and Clarke, K. M.: The pathophysiology of the anterior tibial compartment syndrome: an experimental investigation. J. Trauma 18:299–304, 1978.

Volkmann, R. von: Beiträge zur Chirurgie, Anschliessend an einen Bericht über die Thätigkeit der Chirurgischen. Universitäts Klinik zu Halle in Jahre 1873. Breitkopf & Hartel, Leipzig, 1875, p. 219.

Volkmann, R. von: Die ischaemischen Muskellahmungen und Kontrakturen. Zentralbl. Chir. 8:801–803, 1881.

Volkmann, R. von: Verletzungen und Krankenheiten der Bewegungsorgane. *In* Handbuch der Allgemeinen und Speciellen Chirurgie. F. Enke, Erlangen & Stuttgart, Vol. 2, Pt. 2A, 1882, pp. 234–920.

Whitesides, T. E., Jr., Hirada, H., and Morimoto, K.: The response of skeletal muscle to temporary ischemia: an experimental study. Proc. Am. Acad. Orthop. Surg. J. Bone Joint Surg. 53A:1027–1028, 1971.

Chapter Two

HISTORICAL REVIEW

Steven R. Garfin, M.D.

Clinical awareness of compartment syndromes and their catastrophic sequelae dates back more than a century. Although the entity of Volkmann's ischemic contracture was well known over the last hundred years, the etiology has been less than clear. Phases or eras of "understanding" can be pinpointed to help trace the history of compartment syndromes.

Before 1910 the descriptions by Volkmann were the most influential and emphasized heavily the contracture of the muscles, along with their histologic details. In the early 1900s theories as to the actual development of compartment syndromes, together with clinical descriptions of the acute phase, began appearing in the literature. Murphy (1914) proposed pressure in the subfascial area as the etiologic agent causing ischemia and necrosis. The emphasis, however, changed between 1920 and 1940 when articles by Jepson (1926) and Brooks (1922, 1925, 1934) showed experimentally that venous obstruction was undoubtedly the causative factor. During the years of World War II, Griffiths (1940) and Foisie (1942) espoused the belief that arterial spasm was the sole cause of acute and chronic compartment syndromes, and that all previous authors were in error. In the 1950s and 1960s, however, the cycle returned again to a more descriptive phase involving crush syndromes as well as isolated anterior compartment syndromes of the leg, although at the time these entities were not thought to be related. These eventually were united in etiologic terms after a better understanding of compartment syndromes had developed, and the basic etiology of the syndrome was established as pressure-causing small vessel obstruction and myonecrosis.

CONTRACTURE ERA

Although commonly attributed to Richard von Volkmann, the first actual report of a patient with a presumed ischemic contracture from a compartment syndrome was by Hamilton in 1850. Unfortunately his original description is not available, but it was recorded anecdotally by Hildebrand (1906). To Volkmann, therefore, based on his clear and descriptive analyses, as well as the lack of any previous documentation, is accorded the honor of having drawn attention to the pathologic process of

6

ischemic contractures of the extremities. In deference to his original descriptions, the entity of a residual ischemic contracture from a compartment syndrome is today commonly referred to by the eponym "Volkmann's contracture."

Volkmann (1839–1889) (Fig. 2–1) was born in Leipzig, Germany, where he became Professor of Surgery at the Halle Clinic. He was most noted by his contemporaries for his studies on cancer, and also was credited with introducing the listerian antiseptic techniques to Germany. He was apparently one of the foremost surgeons of the locale, was respected as an educator, and founded an important medical monograph series entitled "Sammlung Klinischen Vortrage." Interestingly, though, he is remembered for his famous work in compartment syndromes and ischemic contractures. According to a biographic review by Talbott (1970), *Volkmann's Ischaemic Paralysis and Contractures* (1881) constitutes one of his lesser contributions but perhaps his best known.

Aside from his medical and surgical work, Volkmann was also a most popular poet of his period under the pen name Richard Leander. He wrote many publicly acclaimed pieces, but his most famous and most quoted poetic works come from his series *The Reveries at French Firesides*. Titles such as *The Rusted Knight*, *The Invisible Kingdom*, and *How The Devil Fell Into The Holy Water* are considered German children's classics and have been translated into English (1908).

Volkmann's early contributions in the area of ischemic contractures began modestly with case reports, his first being published in 1869. In these he described

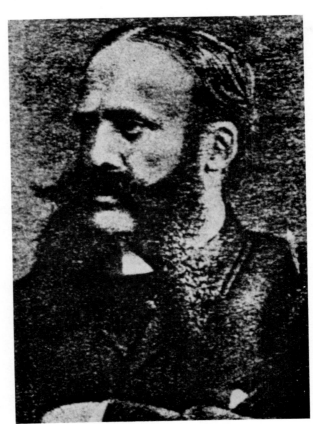

Figure 2–1 Richard von Volkmann (1830–1889). (From Griffiths, D.: Br. J. Surg. 28:239, 1940.)

the first widely acknowledged cases of what were subsequently known as Volkmann's ischemic contractures. Two of his early descriptions were of patients with forearm fractures who, in follow-up examinations, had developed irreversible contractures of the flexor muscles of the wrist and hand. The first case report (1869), largely forgotten by succeeding generations, was of a 16 year old male who had "hydrops" of the knee and who developed a mild deformity in the ipsilateral ankle after the lower extremity swelling subsided.

Realizing the significance of his early cases and the lack of understanding of the disease process, Volkmann reorganized his data and attempted to analyze and explain the pathogenesis of these contractures. He produced the now classic article on the subject, *Die ischaemischen Muskellahmungen und Kontrakturen (Ischemic muscle paralysis and contractures)* (1881). In this article he expounds on the contracture state and relates it for the first time directly to the ischemic condition created by trauma, fractures, bandaging, and subsequent swelling.

> For many years I have been drawing attention to the fact that the paralysis and contractures of the limbs which sometimes follow bandages applied too tightly do not arise as was assumed to paralysis of the nerves by pressure, but through wholesale and swift disintegration of the contractural substance and the resultant reaction and regeneration. The paralysis and contractures should be understood to have their origin in muscle.
>
> Richard von Volkmann, 1881, as
> translated in Rang, M., *Anthology*
> *of Orthopedics.*

Volkmann elucidated many points in his article. Briefly, paraphrasing a few of what we consider to be his most significant points of emphasis:

(1) paralysis and contractures can occur after too tight bandaging;

(2) these changes can develop in either the upper or lower extremities;

(3) the muscle paralysis is secondary to ischemic necrosis and is similar to rigor mortis;

(4) this deformity can be differentiated from strictly nerve palsy by the simultaneous or close onset of paralysis and contracture in the former, and the more gradual development of contractions in the latter;

(5) the degree of contracture increases with time, as does the quantity of the scarred tissue; and

(6) Once the contracture is established, only surgery can salvage the extremity.

Volkmann essentially opened the door to an entity that was seen but poorly understood. His clinical impressions and interpretations were impressive, and he laid the groundwork for further work in this area. Unfortunately, his emphasis on tight bandaging and arterial insufficiency as a primary cause of the contractures was not totally accurate, and may have detracted from the overall significance of his contribution.

Leser, a contemporary of Volkmann, although perhaps not as well known, is credited by many medical historians in the field as being nearly equal to Volkmann in terms of advancing the knowledge of compartment syndromes and ischemic contractures. In fact, in the early literature, the ischemic contracture condition was called by some the "Leser-Volkmann ischaemic contracture" (Thomas, 1909). Leser (1884), like Volkmann, reported several clinical cases of ischemic contractures, but more importantly, he described his investigations on the effect of ischemia in dog, rabbit, and frog limbs as well as the histopathology of the contracted compartment. In examining both the clinical and experimental muscle tissue, he was the first to describe the increased connective tissue pattern and loss of intracellular nuclei seen microscopically in the muscles. Leser's findings basically agreed with those of Volkmann. He felt strongly that contractures and paralyses were of primary muscle origin related to decreased oxygen delivery to the muscle. Leser was not as forceful as his contemporary, and did not hypothesize how this state of diminished muscular oxygen (hypoxia) developed, unlike Volkmann who emphasized tight bandaging and arterial insufficiency. As Volkmann had presented the clinical entity, Leser introduced a laboratory model.

The histologic evaluations of Leser led others to attempt to explain the muscle scarring on an inflammatory basis. Petersen (1888) reported a case of a contracted upper extremity that had some return of distal function after an entrapped median nerve in the forearm was released. Petersen felt that this case, demonstrating return of function after release of scarred tissue, offered increased evidence that scarring and inflammation were major factors in the pathology of Volkmann's ischemic contractures. He also confirmed the microscopic findings observed and reported by Leser. His conclusion was arterial occlusion was a precipitating event leading to muscle ischemia and scarring, and the resultant nerve entrapment and damage. In contrast to Volkmann's primary emphasis, which was on the muscle, Petersen drew some attention to the nerve as one of the systems creating the contracted state.

Up to this time most authors had evaluated the contracture process at one point in its course. Bernays (1900) added to our knowledge by taking a more longitudinal look, and helped develop a picture of the natural history of the ischemic contracture state. He reported the histologic picture in both recently diagnosed and chronic cases of Volkmann's contracture. In the earlier stages he observed that the muscle fibers were irregularly arranged and had unequal thicknesses. In many bundles there was a noticeable absence of nuclei, an abundance of vacuoles, and loss of transverse striations. This is, of course, characteristic of necrotic myofibrils intermittently arranged in relationship to their motor units. Looking at an intermediate stage involving more contraction or chronicity, Bernays noted numerous round cells (lymphocytes and monocytes), increased connective tissue, and decreased muscle cell size. Finally, at the end stage of the disease process, he found marked atrophy and complete disappearance of muscle fibers in his biopsy sections.

Edington (1903) made similar observations to those of Bernays, but found in the same individual, and in fact in the same muscle, the entire spectrum of stages described by Bernays. This discovery at the time was curious; however, it is not necessarily conflicting, as we now know that different degrees of ischemia may develop in adjacent motor units. Later, Rowlands (1905) reported a histologic picture similar to that described both by Bernays and Edington, but he also emphasized that increased interstitial fibrosis was present in the muscle in all stages of the disease, reaffirming the inflammatory nature of the process. Step by step a more complete description was developing.

In the early 1900s, case reports began giving way to more elaborate reviews as well as more detailed laboratory research. Volkmann's contributions were widely known and accepted, although his emphasis on arterial injury and muscle damage did not carry through for the remainder of the century. Twenty years after Volkmann's article, Wallis (1901) wrote that neurologic damage and scarring initiated by hyperemia was the critical feature in creating Volkmann's contracture.

Table 2-1 SUMMARY OF IMPORTANT ASPECTS OF THOMAS' REVIEW
(1909)

Cases Reviewed	112
Sex Distribution	3 male: 1 female
Age	66 cases $\leq$ 15 years old 41 cases $\geq$ 16 years old
Extremities Involved	Upper—107 Lower—5
Predominant Symptoms and Signs	Pain, direct muscle tenderness, immediate postinjury swelling, trophic changes (cyanosis, coldness, shiny skin)

Etiology	Upper Extremities:
	   fractures 91
	   contusions 6
	   bandage/splints 3
	   rest ("quiet") 3
	   embolus 4
	
	Lower Extremities:
	   fractures 1
	   "hydrops" 1
	   ruptured popliteal artery 1
	   embolus 1
	   surgical injury 1

Hildebrand (1906), a student of Volkmann's, agreed with his mentor that damage to the muscle was the primary cause of the contracture, but he felt that nerve contusion and scarring were also factors leading to the poor prognosis. Hildebrand also noted that elevated pressure may be significant in the etiology of ischemic contractures. He considered that an increased venous effusion created an increased pressure in the muscle that subsequently compromised the small arteries and retarded the development of collateral circulation. As will be noted, this is a recurring theme that was given little attention until the 1970s. Perhaps as important as his contributions regarding the etiology of Volkmann's contracture, however, was the fact that Hildebrand was the first to describe this condition in the literature using the eponym "Volkmann's ischemic contracture."

Bardenheuer's (1906) writing at the same time as Hildebrand related the ischemic state to arterial wall injury. He did not believe, however, that arterial wall damage was the sole cause of the contracture but thought that venous stasis and edema were also significant components in the massive inflammatory reaction that developed. He also believed that a build-up of toxic metabolites developed when the venous return was compromised, and that this was the catalyst for the inflammatory process. It was this theory that led Bardenheuer to suggest that a release of these "toxins" through surgical decompression (fasciotomy) might be a most important step in the treatment of this relentless process.

As the history is reviewed, one sees the development of a variety of ideas and reports relating to Volkmann's ischemic contracture. Thomas (1909) took on the formidable task of assimilating all the accumulated data. In a 40-page article, Thomas presented an extensive review of literature on the ischemic contracture process, encompassing and attempting to summarize all the evidence presented up to that time. He did a masterful and complete job, and his article on the early works relating to Volkmann's contracture makes excellent reading. Table 2–1 summarizes only the most important points of Thomas' review.

PRESSURE THEORIES

By 1910 the authorities in the field had proposed many treatment alternatives for the established contractures. It is significant that up to this time the emphasis had been primarily on the contracture itself, and not on the early diagnosis or on preventing the changes from developing.

One of the common suppositions at this time was that the tight bandaging that was frequently applied following fractures or contusions compromised the arterial supply of the extremity. Rowlands (1910) changed this etiologic emphasis by proposing that part of the pressure build-up, and therefore ischemic period, actually occurred after bandage removal. He suggested that, after the release of this circumferential dressing (and therefore obstruction), the blood would return rapidly into the extremity, causing congestion and edema (the edema being caused by the flow of fluid out through overburdened and damaged vessels — a concept in essence identical to present-day beliefs regarding postrevascularization procedures in ischemic limbs, e.g., bypass grafts, embolectomies, and so forth).

Murphy (1914) agreed with Rowlands and suggested that "internal tension" may be the prime consideration. He pointed out that following a fracture blood and serum exuded subfascially and created a significant pressure under tension.

As a result of a fracture . . . blood and serum effusion follows and the tension in the subfascial zone in the forearm can be so great as to cause cyanosis of the whole forearm and hand . . . a blood clot forms in the tissues, inflammation follows with a deposit of the inflammatory products in the tissue . . . it is the pressure which causes the cell destruction.

J.B. Murphy, 1914.

Murphy attributed the inflammatory reaction to the natural sequence of events that follows hemorrhage and necrotic debris accumulating and filling the intracompartmental spaces. His "radical" treatment for this problem was to intercede with fasciotomy before the contracture state developed. He described releasing the forearm fascia from the anterolateral aspect of the arm if symptoms (cyanosis, coolness, pain) persisted. This paper is one of the earliest published that advocates prevention of the contracture state rather than delayed reconstructive treatment. Murphy also described lower extremity compartment syndromes caused by Buck's traction, circular plaster, and compression splints. As noted prior to this time lower extremity compartment syndromes had been merely described in case reports without any particular attention being directed to them. With his concepts on pressure, fasciotomy, and lower extremity involvement, Murphy displayed an unusual understanding of the topic and the significant events leading to the condition of Volkmann's ischemic contracture — at least as we perceive them today.

VENOUS THEORIES

For the next two to three decades the thrust in the study of compartment syndromes was centered around finding a vascular etiology for the disease process.

Both sides of the vascular tree (arterial and venous) were looked at and supported as the primary cause by different authors. Brooks was the first to examine the problem systematically. His emphasis was on the venous side of the system, and he worked hard to develop an experimental compartment syndrome model based on venous occlusion. In an extensive work published in 1922, Brooks looked at both arterial and venous obstruction as possible causes for Volkmann's ischemic contracture. He concluded that, following temporary arterial occlusion, intramuscular hemorrhage and swelling, along with necrosis of muscle fibers, could develop. However, the woody fibrosis and inflammation that clinically accompany the contracture were not routinely observed in this model. Brooks also noted that the extent and duration of the temporary obstruction to arterial flow was critical, and this was difficult to relate to the clinical state. If the ischemia persisted too long, gangrene resulted, but if the obstruction was minimal, recovery could be complete. He was unable to reduplicate the clinical setting consistently.

Exploration of the venous side of the vascular system, however, provided more reproducible results. Brooks discovered he could repeatedly reproduce the hard, ropy, inflammatory condition found in Volkmann's contracture by creating prolonged obstruction of the veins, while leaving the arteries patent. Based on these studies, he concluded that the true etiology of compartment syndromes and ischemic contractures was related to venous outflow obstruction.

That the classic picture of Volkmann's ischemic paralysis could only be explained on the basis of acute venous obstruction would seem quite clear . . . In those instances in which a bandage or splint is applied to an extremity . . . and in which there follows in the course of a few hours great pain and cyanosis which make the constriction no longer bearable, and in which removal of the splint is followed by swelling, heat, tenderness and a rapidly developing contracture, one is forced to the assumption that the etiologic factor is either an acute venous obstruction or a temporary pressure anemia followed by reestablishment of circulation to the damaged tissue. The ease with which the former is reproduced experimentally is evidence of its being the most important etiologic factor of contractures ...

Barney Brooks, 1922

Brooks' extensive research efforts (1922, 1925, 1934) were a cornerstone in vascular surgery for many years. Aside from compartment syndromes he published extensively on a variety of vascular problems during the early 1900s. He contributed much to the overall knowledge of disease states related to lesions of blood vessels, and to this day his work is well respected.

Following Brooks, Jepson (1926), in his master's thesis from the University of Minnesota, Mayo Clinic, analyzed the ischemic contracture process in both the clinical and experimental settings. He, too, concluded that the only experimental models that would accurately reproduce the Volkmann picture involved large vein occlusions or tight bandaging. Like Brooks, he employed dogs in an attempt to develop a venous occlusion model both by direct surgical intervention and with an externally applied tourniquet.

Jepson's other significant contribution, similar to Murphy's 12 years earlier, related to the role of fascia in enveloping and containing intracompartmental pressure. To relieve this increased pressure and perhaps prevent untoward sequelae, Jepson performed fasciotomy in his dogs.

The lesion of ischemic paralysis as seen in humans was reproduced in animals by bandaging one extremity and by preventing the return of venous blood. During attempts to avoid the development of the deformity, it was found that if drainage was instituted within a few hours after the procedures leading to the development of the lesion were performed, contracture either did not ensue or was very slight. The results of these experiments would seem to indicate that the contracture deformity is due to a combination of factors, the most important of which are impairment of the venous flow, extravasation of blood and serum, and swelling of the tissues, with consequent pressure on the blood vessels and nerves in the involved area. If this is true, early drainage (fasciotomy) would be of value.

However, despite this laboratory evidence implicating increased pressure and venous obstruction in compartment syndromes, Jepson was unable to explain fully by his model all the findings associated with clinical compartment syndromes. Therefore, in dealing with actual human cases of Volkmann's ischemic contracture, specifically those of the forearm and hand, he evoked the theory of direct trauma to the ulnar nerve as the primary factor leading to the intrinsic contracture that developed following significant injury.

ARTERIAL THEORIES

After World War II began, a new set or mode of injuries was introduced. Bullet and shrapnel wounds, crush injuries, and other significant massive trauma became common occurrences. Volkmann's ischemic contractures apparently were being seen more often, and new emphasis was laid on the understanding and prevention of the catastrophic processes. Griffiths (1940) and Foisie (1942) felt strongly that previous authors were mistaken in their experimental models, and that the true etiology of Volkmann's ischemia was arterial spasm.

Based upon observations derived from 32 cases, evidence is produced in support of the theory that Volkmann's ischaemic contracture is due to arterial injury and to the accompanying spasm of the collateral circulation. This view is supported by clinical signs of arterial occlusion in acute and chronic cases.

D. L. Griffiths, 1940.

Volkmann's ischemic contracture should be divorced from its association with supracondylar fracture of the humerus. It is the result of a nearly complete ischemia produced by arterial spasm of the main artery and the collateral circulation. Interruption of the sympathetic reflex arc is the rational treatment. Arterectomy gives the best result in stubborn cases.

P. S. Foisie, 1942.

This, then, was the direction taken in the 1940s. All fractures and injuries that showed early signs of ischemic paralysis or involvement were considered by many individuals to need surgical exploration. Griffiths' "four P's" were established to help in the diagnosis of compartment syndromes: (1) pain in the forearm with passive stretch; (2) painless onset; (3) pallor; and (4) pulselessness. If direct arterial injury could not be demonstrated at the time of surgery, many of the surgeons in this period demanded further exploration to uncover the area of arterial spasm. They emphasized that areas of spasm must exist and should be excised before the spasm produced enough ischemia to make the process irreversible. These workers, frequently military surgeons seeing high velocity injuries, "found areas of spasm," performed arterectomies and reanastomoses, and in some cases observed relief of the presurgical ischemic state. In retrospect, it may have been the extensive exploration and fascial release that was necessary that helped relieve the often relentless course of the disease. Perhaps some of these theories will still prove correct, and they should not be completely dismissed. However, at least for that time, Griffiths and his contemporaries completely set aside the earlier research developments and clinical observations.

LEG COMPARTMENT SYNDROMES

The military experience also focused attention on compartment syndromes of the lower extremity. Numerous articles appeared describing "march fractures" and acute anterior tibial syndromes in military recruits. Sirbu et al. (1944), Horn (1945), Vogt (1945), and Hughes (1948) reported a number of anterior leg compartment syndromes that developed in individuals performing strenuous physical activities. These authors proposed that the best treatment was fasciotomy of the leg, to help reverse or prevent neuromuscular damage to the underlying compartment. These articles did not necessarily relate to Volkmann's ischemic contractures, but the idea and implications were obvious (see Chapter 14).

Over this entire course of history, however, the lower limbs still did not receive the same attention as the upper limbs. Focus on the lower extremity, and concern for limb functional capacity following acute compartment syndromes, may be attributed to Seddon (1966), who published an article on Volkmann's ischemia in the lower extremity. He noted how rarely lower limb problems had been reported in the medical literature — a situation not significantly changed since Thomas' 1909 review in which only five out of 112 compartment syndromes reported were of the lower extremity. Seddon, looking exclusively at lower limb disorders, referred to Ellis (1958), who reported on 343 tibial shaft fractures and noted nine cases of ischemic contracture (an incidence of 2.6 per cent). Obviously this syndrome had been occurring, but was not foremost in the minds of the medical community until Ellis, and later Seddon, emphasized its significance. Since then, the medical literature has documented more and more cases of lower limb compartment syndromes.

It was also over this period that functionally, as well as anatomically, the leg was considered to have four compartments rather than only one or two bony or neurologic structures. The posterior deep and superficial compartments of the leg were distinguished originally by Seddon, and later by Kelly and Whitesides (1967), in emphasizing the need to perform four compartment fasciotomies of the leg.

CRUSH SYNDROME

The war years also introduced the "crush syndrome" to the medical sphere. Bywaters and Beall (1941) described massively swollen limbs, myonecrosis, renal failure, and often death in patients crushed during the aerial bombardment of London during World War II. In ensuing years it was also noted in coal-mining accidents, and in 1953 Gordon and Newman described a patient who, after prolonged anesthesia in the knee-chest position, had a similar presentation to that of the crush injuries. This patient, after being maintained too long in the knee-chest position, presented with swollen limbs, shock, myoglobinuria, and renal failure.

In the 1960s and 1970s the crush syndrome was not an infrequent disease state, although now it is more frequently associated with drug overdose patients and the resultant prolonged limb compression position that is maintained. In the time of Bywaters and Beall, however, it was felt to be an isolated entity in no way connected with compartment syndromes, or as they were known at that time, with Volkmann's ischemic contracture (see Chapter 11).

CURRENT CONCEPTS

The history of compartment syndromes and the ischemic contracture state has now essentially gone full cycle. We are currently in a period in which the prime pathophysiologic event in compartment syndromes is generally considered to be an elevation in intracompartmental pressure. An unaltered pressure elevation above a critical level can result in irreversible intracompartmental ischemic contractures (Volkmann's). Pressure measurements are now an accepted mode of determining, as well as definitively diagnosing, compartment syndromes; complete fasciotomy is the treatment of choice to prevent Volkmann's contracture and help reverse the changes in muscles and nerves caused by compartmental tamponade or ischemia.

Today, the major discussions and disagreements in the literature are related not so much to etiology or prevention of compartment syndromes, but more to the diagnosis and specific types of decompression. Controversy also exists as to which type of intracompartmental pressure-measuring device is the most accurate and efficient (see Chapter 7).

It was not until the 1970s that the interrelationship of all the preceding entities was firmly established. It then became evident that not only the crush syndrome, presenting with renal failure, shock, severe muscle damage, and necrosis, but also anterior tibial syndromes, Volkmann's ischemia, and compartment syndromes were all similar entities with the same basic pathophysiology and the same end result if untreated — muscle necrosis and contracture resulting in Volkmann's contracture. This final "unified concept" can be credited to the work of Reneman (1968), Matsen (1975), Mubarak and Owen (1975), Rorabeck and MacNab (1975), Sheridan and Matsen (1975), Whitesides et al. (1975), and Mubarak et al. (1976), along with the accumulated experience of all the previously mentioned authors in this field.

REFERENCES

Bardenheuer, L.: Die ischämische Kontraktur und Gangrän als Folge der Arterienverletzung. Leuthold's Gedenkschrift 2:87, 1906.

Bernays, A. C.: On ischemic paralysis and contractures of muscles. Boston Med. Surg. J. 542:539, 1900.

Brooks, B.: Pathologic changes in muscle as a result of disturbances of circulation. Arch. Surg. 5:188, 1922.

Brooks, B.: New methods for study of disease of the circulation of the extremities. J. Bone Joint Surg. 7:316, 1925.

Brooks, B., Johnson, J. S., and Kirtley, J. A.: Simultaneous vein ligation. Surg. Gynecol. Obstet. 59:496, 1934.

Bywaters, E. G. L., and Beall, D.: Crush injuries with impairment of renal function. Br.. Med. J. 1:427, 1941.

Davies-Colley, J. N. C.: Contractures of flexor muscles of forearm following splint pressure. Guy's Hospital Gazette 12:460, 1898.

Edington, G. H.: Tendon lengthening in a case of Volkmann's ischaemic paralysis. Glas. Med. J. 54:344, 1900.

Edington, G. H.: Volkmann's contracture. Glas. Med. J. 59:417, 1903.

Ellis, H.: Disabilities after tibial shaft fractures with special reference to Volkmann's ischaemic contracture. J. Bone Joint Surg. 40B:190, 1958.

Foisie, P. S.: Volkmann's ischemic contracture: an analysis of its approximate mechanism. N. Engl. J. Med. 226:671, 1942.

Gordon, B. S., and Newman, W.: Lower nephron syndrome following prolonged knee-chest position. J. Bone Joint Surg. 35-A:764, 1953.

Griffiths, D.: Volkmann's ischaemic contracture. Br. J. Surg. 28:239, 1940.

Guyton, A. C.: A concept of negative interstitial pressure based on pressures in implanted perforated capsules. Circ. Res. 12:399, 1963.

Hildebrand, O.: Die Lehre von den ischämische Muskellahmungen und Kontrakturen. Samml. Klin. Vortrage 122:437, 1906.

Holmes, W., Highet, W. V., and Seddon, H. J.: Ischaemic nerve lesions occurring in Volkmann's contracture. Br. J. Surg. 32:259, 1944.

Horn, C. E.: Acute ischemia of the anterior tibial muscle and the long extensor muscles of the toes. J. Bone Joint Surg. 27-A:615, 1945.

Hughes, J. R.: Ischaemic necrosis of the anterior tibial muscles due to fatigue. J. Bone Joint Surg. 30-B:581, 1948.

Jepson, P. N.: Ischemic contracture — experimental study. Ann. Surg. 84:785, 1926.

Kelly, R. P., and Whitesides, T. E., Jr.: Transfibular route for fasciotomy of the leg. J. Bone Joint Surg. 49A:1022, 1967.

Kjellmer, I.: An indirect method for estimating tissue pressure with special reference to tissue pressure and muscle joint exercise. Acta Physiol. Scand. 62:31, 1964.

Landerer, A.: Die Gewebsspannung in ihrem Einfluss auf die Ortliche Blut-und Lymphbewegung. C. W. Vogel, Leipzig, 1884.

Leander, R.: Reveries at French Firesides. Ginn and Co., New York, 1908.

Leser, E.: Untersuchungen uber ischämische Muskellahmungen und Muskelkontrakturen. Samml. Klin. Vortrage 249, 1884.

Littlewood, H.: Some complications following injuries about the elbow joint and their treatment. Lancet 1:290, 1900.

Matsen, F. A.: Compartmental syndrome: a unified concept. Clin. Orthop. 113:8, 1975.

Mubarak, S. J., Hargens, A. R., Owen, C. A., Garetto, L. P., and Akeson, W. H.: The wick catheter technique for measurement of intramuscular pressure: a new research and clinical tool. J. Bone Joint Surg. 58-A:1016, 1976.

Mubarak, S. J., and Owen, C. A.: Compartment syndrome and its relation to the crush syndrome: a spectrum of disease. Clin. Orthop. 113:81, 1975.

Murphy, J. B.: Myositis. J. A. M. A. 63:1249, 1914.

Petersen, F.: Ueber ischämische Muskellahmungen. Arch. Klin. Chir. 37:675, 1888.

Reneman, R. S.: The anterior and lateral compartment syndrome of the leg. Mouton, The Hague, Paris, 1968.

Rorabeck, C. H., and MacNab, I.: The pathophysiology of the anterior tibial compartmental syndrome. Clin. Orthop. 113:52, 1975.

Rowlands, R. P.: A case of Volkmann's contracture treated by shortening the radius and ulna. Lancet 2:1168, 1905.

Rowlands, R. P.: Volkmann's contracture. Guy's Hosp. Gaz. 24:87, 1910.

Seddon, H. J.: Volkmann's ischaemia in the lower limb. J. Bone Joint Surg. 48B:627, 1966.

Sheridan, G. W., and Matsen, F. A.: An animal model of the compartmental syndrome. Clin. Orthop. 113:36, 1975.

Sirbu, A. B., Murphy, M. J., and White, A. S.: Soft tissue complications of fractures of the leg. Calif. West. Med. 60:1, 1944.

Talbott, J. H.: A Biographical History of Medicine. Grune and Stratton, New York, 1970.

Thomas, J. J.: Nerve involvement in the ischaemic paralysis and contracture of Volkmann. Ann. Surg. 49:330, 1909.

Vogt, P. R.: Ischemic muscular necrosis following marching. Read before the Oregon State Medical Society, Sept. 4, 1943 (cited by Horn, C.E., 1945).

Volkmann, R. von: Krankenheiten der Bewegungsorgane. In Handbuch der Chirurgie (Pitha-Billroth). Erlangen 2:846, 1869.

Volkmann, R. von: Die ischaemischen Muskellahmungen und Kontrakturen. Zentralbl. Chir. 8:801, 1881.

Wallis, F. C.: Treatment of paralysis and muscular atrophy after prolonged use of splints or of an Esmarch's cord. Practitioner 67:429, 1901.

Wells, H. S., Youmans, J. B., and Miller, D. G.: Tissue pressure (intercutaneous, subcutaneous and intramuscular) as related to venous pressure, capillary filtration and other factors. J. Clin. Invest. 17:489, 1939.

Whitesides, T. E., Haney, T. C., Morimoto, K., and Harada, H.: Tissue pressure measurements as a determinant for the need of fasciotomy. Clin. Orthop. 113:43, 1975.

Chapter Three

ANATOMY OF THE EXTREMITY COMPARTMENTS

Steven R. Garfin, M.D.

INTRODUCTION

An anatomic compartment consists primarily of the muscles, arteries, veins, and nerves confined within a relatively closed osseofascial space (Fig. 3–1). Whether the boundaries are strictly fascial or a combination of fascia and bone is incidental to this definition. The muscles in a compartment tend to act as a functional unit, whereas the nerves and arteries frequently are only coinhabitants as they course through the compartment on their way to their more distal, ultimate destination.

Employing the above criteria for this chapter, the human body can be divided into numerous compartments — many with multiple, but some with only single, muscle components.

The purpose of this chapter is not to elaborate in great detail on all of these compartments and their anatomic contents, since adequate information of this kind can be found in most anatomy textbooks. Our concern is rather with the motor or functional elements more frequently involved in compartment syndromes. The focus of this section, therefore, will be predominantly on these areas and the possible functional consequences of increased pressure developing in one of these units. Only the more salient features of the commonly involved regions will be described, and an attempt will be made to correlate this anatomic information with the clinical findings.

GENERAL DESCRIPTIONS

Fascia

Fascia is a dense, regular, connective tissue associated with, but distinct from, the underlying muscles. In some cases the muscle may originate from the overlying fascia. In others the epimysium and fascia may be adherent, forming one unit. For the most part, however, the fascia and the epimysium are structurally separate entities.

COMPONENTS OF A GENERALIZED
MUSCLE COMPARTMENT

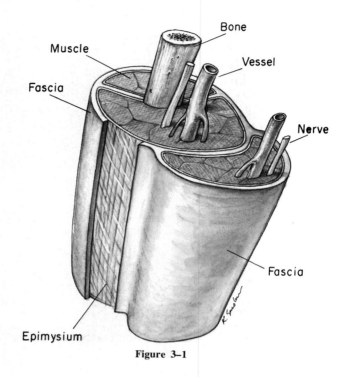

Figure 3–1

Fascia is composed of collagenous bundles and fibroblasts arranged in sheets, each with fairly parallel, wave-like rows of collagen. Fibers from one sheet interweave with adjoining layers and contribute to the overall strength of the completed structure. Although the histology is well known, the biomechanics and "function" of the fascia are poorly understood. It has been shown, however, that the investing (or containing) role of fascia does enhance the power of the underlying muscle; and removing the fascia reduces the force of underlying muscle contractions by nearly 15 per cent (Garfin et al., 1981). This apparently occurs secondary to a reduction of the volume-containing ability of the compartment itself, probably allowing the muscle to balloon out and thereby losing contractile efficiency.

Muscles

Muscles act variously in the body to help stabilize, accelerate, or decelerate body parts (Basmajian, 1967). Just as the function varies from muscle to muscle, so do the individual characteristics. Some muscles work primarily through a single joint, whereas others cross multiple joints. Contractile and performance efficiency also are determined by the shape and fascicular pattern of the muscle (Fig. 3–2). The strength characteristic is partially related to the configuration and direction of the muscle fibers relative to the direction of contraction of the muscle (Bourne, 1960).

In general terms (Fig. 3–2), the most superficial layer of a muscle is termed the epimysium. This is a connective tissue layer encasing the individual muscle fibers into a larger functional unit. The epimysium in some areas may be firmly attached or fused to the overlying fascia, and in those situations acts as a very thick, strong, structural envelope. Connective tissue septa run from the epimysium through the structure of the muscle to separate the muscle into individual fascicles (Fig. 3–2). Running along the septa is a fine, intertwined meshwork of capillaries and nerves that eventually invaginate the myofibrils to the level of the individual muscle fiber and surrounding sarcolemma. The connective tissue septa themselves, however, do not actually penetrate the thin cellular wall (sarcolemma).

Individual muscle fibers, even within the same fascicles, do not necessarily have a uniform length. Some fibers extend the entire length of the muscle, and some interweave or interdigitate with other, shorter structures to form the entire unit.

As noted previously, the significant factor in the strength of the muscle is the orientation of the fibers to the longitudinal axis of the muscle itself. To help categorize muscles according to shape and function, different types have been grouped together (Fig. 3–3). One group of muscles is described as having a parallel or fusiform pattern where the individual muscle fibers essentially run in a relatively straight line from origin to insertion. Another group, termed unipinnate, have the muscle fibers oriented oblique to the axis of contraction. These muscles have a tendinous origin eccentrically located with respect to the muscle mass. Bipinnate and multipinnate muscles tend to have fibers oriented in a crisscrossing pattern, and in these cases the tendon arises centrally as the various fibers converge on the longitudinal axis. In these muscles, owing to the meshed nature of the muscle fibers them-

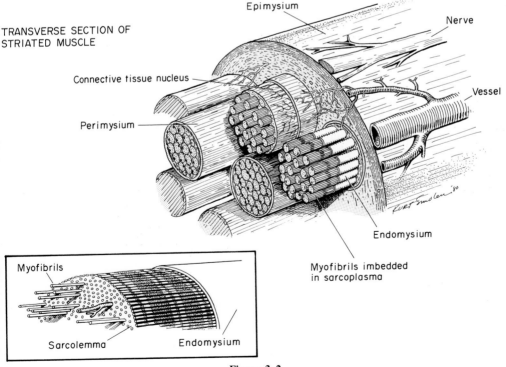

TRANSVERSE SECTION OF STRIATED MUSCLE

Epimysium

Nerve

Connective tissue nucleus

Vessel

Perimysium

Endomysium

Myofibrils

Myofibrils imbedded in sarcoplasma

Sarcolemma

Endomysium

Figure 3–2

MUSCLE TYPES

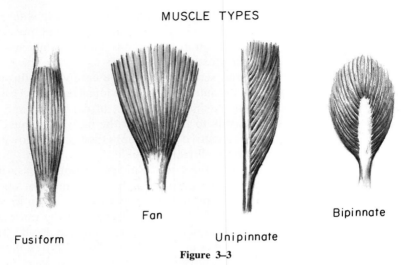

Fusiform   Fan   Unipinnate   Bipinnate

Figure 3–3

selves (Huber, 1916), the connective tissue septa also become intermixed and actually may tightly compartmentalize each muscle unit within the overall pattern (Fig. 3–4).

Nerves

Nerves may be considered miniature compartments, consisting of large bundles of fasciculi (Fig. 3–5). The bundles are grouped and encased in surrounding epineurium. Individually these bundles are enveloped by perineurium. Within the perineurium the nerve fasciculi are further subdivided by endoneurial sheets. Therefore, examining separately each fascicle, one sees a minicompartment with circumferential perineurium (connective tissue) surrounding organized nerve fibers, as well as their nutrient arterioles, capillaries, and venules (compare to muscle).

In the model presented (Rydevik and Lundborg, 1977; Sunderland, 1978), any venous stasis along or within the epineurial sheet, or increased external pressure on the peripheral nerve itself, may be reflected by engorgement within the confines of the perineurial envelope. This process could then obstruct arteriolar inflow and lead to ischemia of the nerve fibers, with subsequent loss of function (similar to a compartment syndrome at the more gross and obvious osseofascial level).

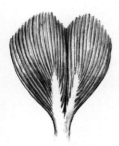

Figure 3–4   Multipinnate muscle.

Multipinnate

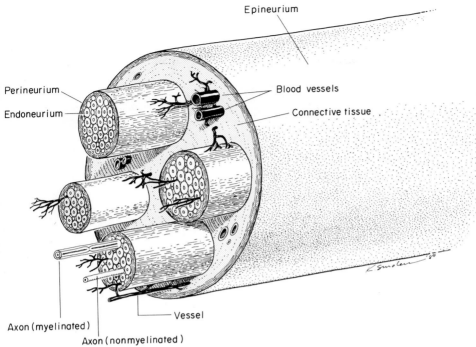

Epineurium

Perineurium

Endoneurium

Blood vessels

Connective tissue

Vessel

Axon (myelinated)

Axon (nonmyelinated)

Figure 3–5 Transverse section of a nerve.

Vascular System

ARTERIES

Knowledge of the smaller, peripheral, vascular bed structures (Fig. 3–6) is important to the understanding of compartment syndromes. Briefly, after leaving the mainstem artery the efferent circulatory system branches into smaller and smaller, muscularly-walled precapillaries or arterioles. Arterioles can then lead directly to venules through arteriovenous anastomoses (thin-walled arterioles containing contractile smooth muscle for control of shunting). More frequently, however, arterioles channel into precapillaries and then capillaries that connect to the venules and larger venous system. Fine tuning of the systemic blood pressure can be controlled by the small, muscularly-walled vessels as well as by shunting blood through collateral channels around the capillary bed (Fig. 3–7). The pressures in capillaries of skeletal muscle range between 20 and 30 mm Hg. Therefore, external pressures that exceed this value may occlude these capillaries that deliver oxygen and remove carbon dioxide during normal blood flow. It is at this microvascular level that increased interstitial fluid pressure first affects compartmental contents and leads to the progressive pathology found in compartment syndromes.

Similar to the varying types of muscles, different patterns of blood supply within the muscles have been described. According to Blomfield (1945), muscles in general have isolated vascular support systems with limited internal and external anastomoses, and therefore anatomic relationships may be inconstant. In some muscles abundant communications between arteriolar systems exist (longitudinal anasto-

ARTERY　　　　　　　　　　　　　　　　　　　　　　　　VEIN

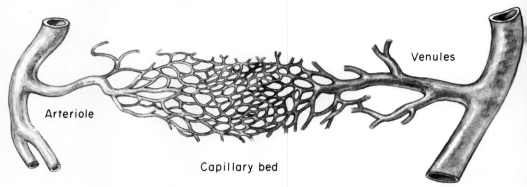

Figure 3–6　Peripheral vascular structures.

motic chains: e.g., soleus and peroneus longus); in others, several mainstem arteries send arterial branches into the muscle so that damage to a single vessel may not be critical (e.g., anterior tibialis and flexor hallucis longus). Some, however, have a single blood supply with few anastomoses (radiating patterns: e.g., biceps; or quadrilateral patterns: e.g., extensor hallucis longus). These latter systems are extremely susceptible to any circulatory compromise by virtue of their single vascular stem (Clark and Blomfield, 1945; Saunders et al., 1957). Edwards (1946) noted that tendons have for the most part a substantial and fairly constant blood supply that may form an anastomosis with the muscular system. He also felt that the vascularity of muscles may be isolated from surrounding tissue and, therefore, susceptible to arterial injury. Wollenberg (1905) earlier described numerous anas-

COLLATERAL CIRCULATION

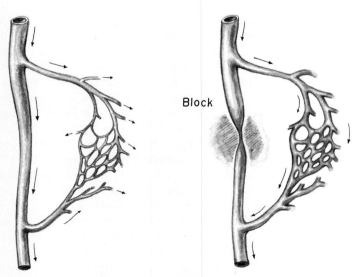

Figure 3–7　Collateral circulation of the peripheral vessels.

tomoses between the vascular system of the tendon and the associated muscle arcades, but noted that the anastomoses were scant and probably not significant in an acute ischemic episode.

VEINS

The venous system as a discrete entity will not be dealt with in this chapter. In general, every major artery in a limb has one or two veins traveling with it, and these will not be specified. This, however, is not to downplay the importance of the venous system. Theoretically, any stasis or engorgement in this system may retard blood flow, causing increased pressure in the small arteriolar capillary system and leading to an alteration in the Starling equilibrium (see Chapter 4). This could then cause fluid extrusion from the capillary walls, and perhaps add to, or create, increased pressure in a closed compartment.

Two other points should be emphasized regarding this system. First, since the venous walls are thinner and less muscular than comparable arterial channels, they are more compressible and therefore more susceptible to changes in surrounding muscle and interstitial fluid pressure. Second, the extremities have essentially two venous flow networks, the superficial and the deep. Deep veins are apparently more efficient in maintaining blood flow. Through the forces of external muscular pumping and the system of intimal valves and communicating branches, blood is predominantly shunted to, and transported through, the deep vessels. These two facts become important in relation to compartment syndrome etiologies (see Chapter 5 — Phlegmasia cerulea dolens).

COMPARTMENTS

Deltoid Compartment

ANATOMY

The boundaries of this compartment are composed primarily of the investing fascia of the deltoid muscle, except for the posteromedial wall, which is supported by the humerus. The deltoid muscle is the sole muscular component of this compartment (Fig. 3–8). The blood supply is derived from the deltoid branch of the thoracoacromial artery and from the posterior humeral circumflex artery, which branches off the axillary artery and passes with the axillary nerve into the compartment through the quadrangular space around the surgical neck of the humerus. The muscle is innervated by the axillary nerve, which therefore is also contained within the compartment. Along with this nerve, the upper lateral brachial cutaneous nerve (a sensory branch of the axillary) may pass through the compartment, and supply sensation to the lateral portion of the shoulder and the skin overlying the deltoid muscle.

CLINICAL CORRELATION

Tenderness, tenseness, or localized erythema without evidence of infection over the deltoid muscle may be associated with an underlying compartment

CIRCUMFLEX BRANCH OF
AXILLARY N.

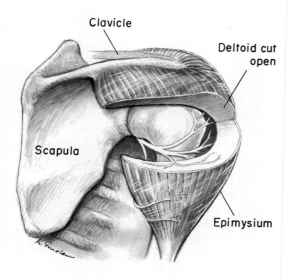

Clavicle

Deltoid cut
open

Scapula

Epimysium

Figure 3–8 Deltoid compartment (posterior view): the epimysium and fascia form one layer enclosing this muscle.

COMPARTMENT
STRUCTURES
OF UPPER ARM

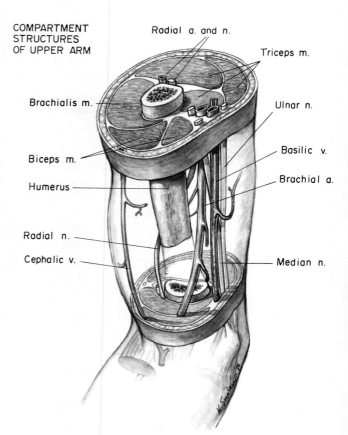

Radial a. and n.

Triceps m.

Brachialis m.

Ulnar n.

Basilic v.

Biceps m.

Brachial a.

Humerus

Radial n.

Cephalic v.

Median n.

Figure 3–9 The biceps-brachialis (anterior) and triceps (posterior) compartments of the right arm.

syndrome. Other associated findings may be diminished active abduction of the shoulder or shoulder pain with passive adduction. Hypoesthesia over the superior lateral aspect of the brachium, consistent with involvement of the upper lateral brachial cutaneous nerve, may also be detected on specific examination of the region.

Arm: Biceps–Brachialis or Anterior Compartment

ANATOMY

The brachial fascia, a continuation of the deltoid fascia, covers this compartment anteriorly, and firmly attaches at its distal extent to the medial and lateral epicondyles of the humerus (Figs. 3–9, 3–10). The medial and lateral walls are formed by the medial intermuscular and lateral intermuscular septa, respectively. The septa join to the posterior wall — the humerus — and terminate distally at the supracondylar ridges. The predominant muscular contents of this compartment are the biceps, brachialis, and coracobrachialis muscles. The mobile wad (brachioradialis and extensors carpi radialis longus and brevis muscles) takes origin in the distal

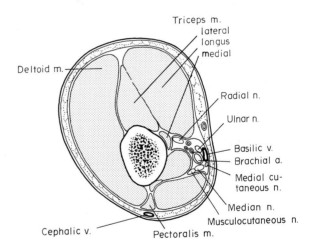

Figure 3–10 Arm compartments: transverse sections through the proximal and distal third of the right arm.

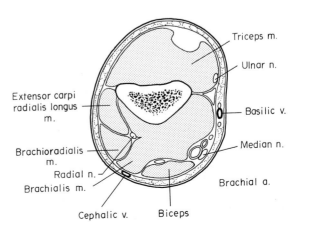

aspect, but generally is not included in this group. The biceps and brachialis, the major muscles in the compartment, are innervated by the musculocutaneous nerve. They have a common arterial supply from the brachial artery.

Along with the brachial artery, the other major vessel in the biceps-brachialis compartment is the basilic vein, which penetrates the brachial fascia in the middle third of the arm. The nerves in this compartment are the median and ulnar nerves, the musculocutaneous nerve, and the lateral antebrachial cutaneous nerve, which is a sensory continuation of the musculocutaneous nerve to the lateral volar aspect of the forearm. Except for the musculocutaneous nerve motor supply, the nerves located here primarily share space as they traverse distally to the forearm and hand. The radial nerve, though primarily a posterior (triceps) compartment nerve, enters the biceps-brachialis compartment through the lateral intermuscular septum in the distal third of the arm, and remains lateral to the brachialis in its distal extent (Fig. 3–11).

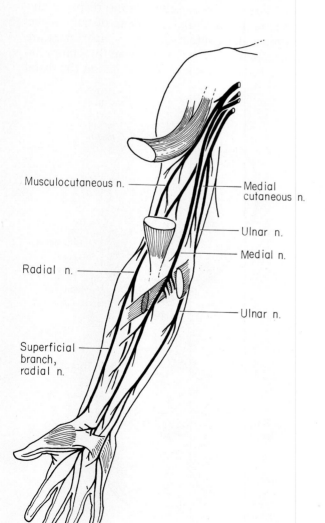

Musculocutaneous n.

Medial cutaneous n.

Ulnar n.

Medial n.

Radial n.

Ulnar n.

Superficial branch, radial n.

Figure 3–11 Nerves of arm and forearm.

CLINICAL CORRELATION

Since the biceps-brachialis compartment acts primarily to flex the elbow, this is the function that would be first affected by a compartment syndrome here. Passive elbow extension would cause pain over the anterior surface of the brachium if significantly elevated pressures were present in this group of muscles. Similarly, weakness in active flexion and tenderness over the biceps and brachialis muscles would be a consistent finding. Paresis in the upper extremity muscles innervated by the median, ulnar, and radial nerves is also a characteristic finding due to ischemia of the nerves as they pass through the biceps-brachialis compartment to their termination in the forearm and hand. Hypoesthesia in the distribution of the median, ulnar, or radial nerves may also be present, as well as diminished sensation over the lateral distal skin of the volar forearm from involvement of the lateral antebrachial cutaneous nerve.

Arm: Triceps or Posterior Compartment

ANATOMY

The deep or brachial fascia extends posteriorly over this compartment. As with the biceps-brachialis compartment, the medial and lateral intermuscular septa to the humerus also limit the triceps. In this case, however, the septa comprise the anterior wall of the compartment (Fig. 3–10). These septa, therefore, separate the anterior from the posterior compartments. The predominant blood supply to the muscle is the profunda brachii artery. The triceps muscle fills this compartment and is innervated by the radial nerve. The radial nerve, the major nerve in the triceps compartment, leaves the compartment through the lateral intermuscular septum in the distal third, and enters the flexor surface. Conversely, on the ulnar side of the arm, in a roughly equivalent transverse plane, the ulnar nerve leaves the biceps-brachialis compartment through the medial intermuscular septum, and associates itself with the triceps group (Fig. 3–10).

CLINICAL CORRELATION

The major function of the triceps muscle — elbow extension — would be compromised with elevated pressures in the triceps compartment. Passive elbow flexion would cause pain posteriorly in the brachium. Hypoesthesia over the dorsum of the hand, which is supplied by the superficial radial nerve, and also along the distribution of the ulnar nerve may be additional findings. Weakness in the muscles innervated by the radial and ulnar nerves, without associated passive stretch pain, may also be noted.

Forearm: Volar Compartment

ANATOMY

Anteriorly, medially, and laterally, this compartment is encased by the antebrachial fascia. This fascia sends strong septal bands to the superficial border of the

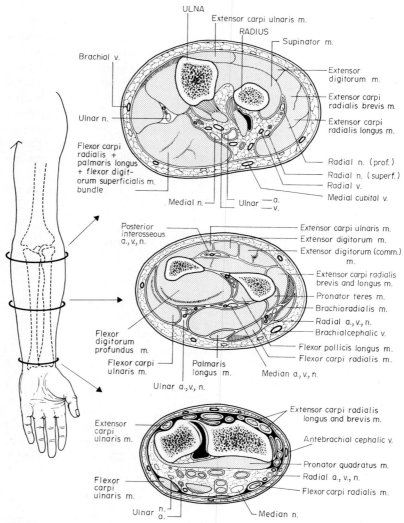

ULNA
Extensor carpi ulnaris m.
RADIUS
Supinator m.
Brachial v.
Extensor digitorum m.
Extensor carpi radialis brevis m.
Extensor carpi radialis longus m.
Ulnar n.
Flexor carpi radialis + palmaris longus + flexor digitorum superficialis m. bundle
Radial n. (prof.)
Radial n. (superf.)
Radial v.
Medial cubital v.
Medial n.
Ulnar a. v.

Posterior interosseous a., v, n.
Extensor carpi ulnaris m.
Extensor digitorum m.
Extensor digitorum (comm.) m.
Extensor carpi radialis brevis and longus m.
Pronator teres m.
Brachioradialis m.
Radial a, v, n.
Brachialcephalic v.
Flexor pollicis longus m.
Flexor carpi radialis m.
Flexor digitorum profundus m.
Flexor carpi ulnaris m.
Palmaris longus m.
Median a, v, n.
Ulnar a., v, n.

Extensor carpi radialis longus and brevis m.
Extensor carpi ulnaris m.
Antebrachial cephalic v.
Pronator quadratus m.
Radial a., v, n.
Flexor carpi radialis m.
Flexor carpi ulnaris m.
Ulnar n. a.
Median n.

Figure 3–12   Forearm compartments: transverse sections through the left forearm at various levels.

ulna and radius. The posterior limits consist of the ulna, radius, and intervening interosseous membrane, along with the septa from bone to antebrachial fascia (Fig. 3–12). In the distal half of the forearm a thinner sheet of fascia extends from medial to lateral, separating the three superficial muscles (palmaris longus, flexor carpi radialis, and flexor carpi ulnaris) from the deeper structures. Proximally, at the entrance of the compartment, the lacertus fibrosus (from the biceps) and the pronator teres create formidable barriers. Distally, the compartment ends at the transverse carpal ligament.

The volar compartment consists essentially of the flexors and pronators of the forearm and wrist. These may be further divided into superficial and deep groups. Beginning at the ulnar border, the superficial muscles are the flexor carpi ulnaris, palmaris longus, flexor carpi radialis, and pronator teres. All these muscles arise at least partially from the common flexor tendon originating at the medial epicondyle of the humerus. The deeper group of muscles consists of the flexor digitorum superficialis and profundus, as well as the flexor pollicis longus, and distally the smaller pronator quadratus. The median nerve supplies most of the muscles in the deep group, except the muscles to the ring and little finger of the flexor digitorum profundus, which are innervated by the ulnar nerve. The median nerve lies between the superficialis and profundus muscles within the superficialis fascia. The anterior interosseous nerve, supplying the long flexors to the thumb and index finger, lies deep to the profundus. The ulnar nerve, coursing with the ulnar artery, is protected superficially by the flexor carpi ulnaris muscle. The blood supply to the muscles, as well as to the hand, is supplied by the ulnar and radial arteries, which are included in the volar forearm compartment.

CLINICAL CORRELATION

The muscles and nerves that lie in the volar forearm compartment function mainly to supply hand and wrist power and control. Elevation of pressure in this compartment, therefore, would affect primarily sensation and motor function on the flexor or palmar surface of the hand (Fig. 3–13). Volar forearm muscle ischemia from a compartment syndrome may be reflected in the hand by decreased strength in the finger and thumb flexors — both deep and superficial. Paresis of the intrinsic muscles would also be noted secondary to involvement of the ulnar and median nerves in the forearm. The fingers may assume a flexed posture owing to some reflex shortening of the forearm muscles. Passive extension of the fingers, causing pain in the volar forearm, would also be indicative of underlying elevated pressures and muscle ischemia in the forearm. Of course, tenseness and tenderness are usually present and located over the volar aspect of the foream.

CUTANEOUS NERVE DISTRIBUTION - HAND

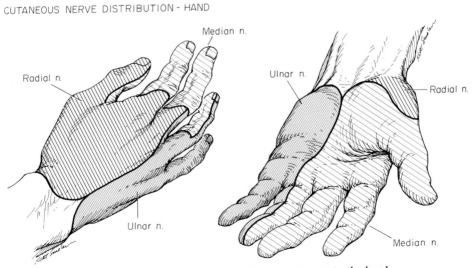

Figure 3–13 Distribution of the cutaneous nerves to the hand.

Forearm: Dorsal Compartment

ANATOMY

As in the volar compartment, the limiting factors are the antebrachial fascia that surrounds the compartment dorsally and to the sides, as well as the ulna and radius and the intervening interosseous membrane anteriorly (Fig. 3–12). The main muscles in this compartment comprise the wrist and finger extensors. The mobile wad (see earlier in this chapter) is physically and functionally located in this group, but is compartmentally separated from the formal contents of the dorsal compartment by separating fascia. The mobile wad, in fact, may be considered a separate compartment, although Gelberman and associates (1978) have shown in terms of surgical decompression that it may be approached along with the volar forearm muscles. The remaining muscles that formally comprise the compartment are the extensor digitorum communis, extensor carpi ulnaris, abductor pollicis longus, and extensors pollicis longus and brevis. The motor units to these latter "outcropper muscles" to the thumb and index finger are supplied by the posterior interosseous nerve. This nerve is the continuation of the radial nerve after it separates from the superficial radial at the supinator muscle. The radial artery lies just volar to the brachioradialis muscle. In the forearm this artery should be considered a member of the volar forearm compartment.

CLINICAL CORRELATION

The dorsal compartment muscles are the functional components for wrist and finger extension. Therefore, elevated intracompartmental pressure in the dorsal forearm could lead to paresis of these extensors, although the hand may assume an extended posture from the extensors acting primarily through the metacarpophalangeal joints. Passive finger or wrist flexion may also generate pain in the involved dorsal compartment muscles. Any sensory deficit may be minimal, as the superficial radial nerve is located primarily in the volar compartment, and may not be routinely affected by dorsal compartment pressure elevations.

Hand Compartments

ANATOMY

The hand can be divided into four structural compartments (Fig. 3–14). These compartments are divided by relatively firm fascia that limits fluid or pressure transmission. They should be differentiated from the potential "spaces" described by Kanavel (1933), composed of loose, filmy, connective tissue, that have been associated with pathways for spread of hand infections (midpalmar and -thenar).

The important, true anatomic compartments related to this monograph are the central palmar, hypothenar, thenar, and interossei.

The *central palmar compartment* is bounded anteriorly by the tough palmar aponeurosis, radially by the thenar septum (attaching posteriorly to the index metacarpal), ulnarly by the hypothenar septum (attaching posteriorly to the fifth

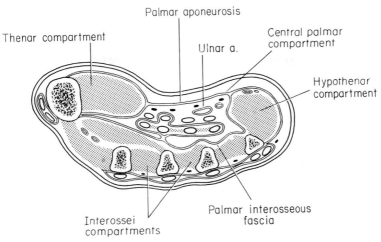

Thenar compartment

Palmar aponeurosis

Ulnar a.

Central palmar compartment

Hypothenar compartment

Interossei compartments

Palmar interosseous fascia

Figure 3–14 Hand compartments: transverse section through the right hand.

metacarpal), and distally by the palmar interosseous fascia that overlies the interossei and adductor pollicis muscles. The central palmar compartment consists primarily of the tendons for the fingers, i.e., flexor digitorum superficialis and profundus, and the lumbricals. The *hypothenar compartment* is bound anteriorly and laterally by the hypothenar fascia (a weaker continuation of the palmar aponeurosis), medially by the hypothenar septum, and posteriorly by the metacarpals. The hypothenar compartment muscles are the abductor digiti minimi, flexor digiti minimi, and opponens digiti minimi. The *thenar compartment* has an anterior or superficial cover consisting of the thenar fascia (similar in consistency to the hypothenar fascia). Its medial and posterior margins are bound by the thenar septum and a lateral bony wall consisting of the thumb metacarpal. The thenar compartment contains the thumb muscles: abductor pollicis brevis, flexor pollicis brevis, opponens, and the tendon of the flexor pollicis longus in its course to the distal phalanx of the thumb. The *interossei* are bound anteriorly by the palmar interosseous fascia, and dorsally by the interosseous fascia. The bony metacarpals complete the compartment side walls. The interossei compartments are separate, and contain the palmar and dorsal interossei to the fingers as well as the adductor pollicis for the thumb.

The common, as well as proper, digital arteries and nerves pass through the central palmar compartment.

CLINICAL CORRELATION

Since the muscles in the four hand compartments are primarily the intrinsics to the hand, these are the functions that would be involved with compartment syndromes. Elevated pressure in the central palmar compartment could cause hypoesthesia on the volar surface of the fingers. Tenseness in the central area of the palm may be remarkable. However, central palmar compartment involvement probably would not demonstrate any significant muscular deficit. The thenar compartment, contrarily, would have markedly demonstrable muscle involvement. A weakness in thumb opposition, as well as limited flexion, may be detectable. Since abductors and flexors exist in the thenar compartment, almost any passive motion may cause pain in the thenar area. Similarly, the hypothenar compartment contains the short abductors, flexors, and opponens to the little finger. Nearly any passive motion of the little finger would cause pain in the hypothenar muscle mass, and limited little finger flexion and abduction may also be demonstrable. Tenseness over these three compartments may also be more obvious than in other compartments of the body. The final hand compartment, consisting of the interossei, is not easy to palpate clinically, and therefore it may be difficult to detect increased pressure easily. Elevated pressure in the interossei would probably create an intrinsic plus hand, with relatively extended interphalangeal joints and a flexed metacarpophalangeal joint. Flexion of the interphalangeal joint would cause pain to, and resistance from, the patient.

These findings should be differentiated from a volar forearm compartment. In the latter instance no tenseness in the hand would be present. Since the nerves to the interossei would be affected, as distinct from the intrinsic muscles themselves, an intrinsic plus deformity probably would not be an early finding. In fact, with ulnar nerve ischemia and dysfunction, an intrinsic minus hand would perhaps be an earlier finding consistent with volar forearm compartment involvement.

Gluteal Compartments

ANATOMY

The muscles contained in this group, as the name implies, are the gluteus maximus, medius, and minimus, as well as the tensor fascia femoris. The gluteal muscles are actually divided into three separate compartments (Fig. 3–15): (1) tensor; (2) medius/minimus; and (3) maximus (Owen et al., 1978). All are at least partially invested by the fascia lata. The fascia lata is attached superiorly to the iliac crest and medially to the sacrum, and laterally it continues into the fascia of the

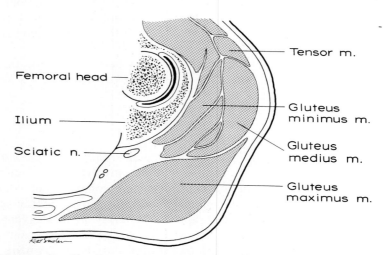

Figure 3–15 Gluteal compartments: transverse section through the gluteal area.

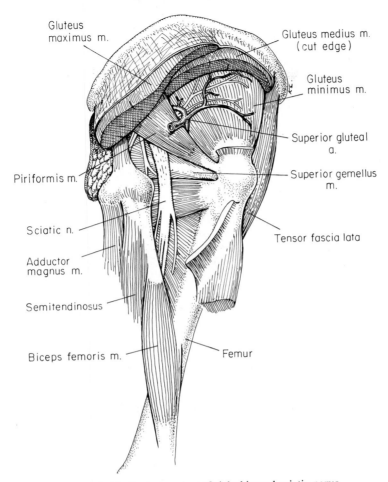

Gluteus maximus m.

Gluteus medius m. (cut edge)

Gluteus minimus m.

Superior gluteal a.

Superior gemellus m.

Piriformis m.

Sciatic n.

Tensor fascia lata

Adductor magnus m.

Semitendinosus

Biceps femoris m.

Femur

Figure 3–16 Posterior view of right hip and sciatic nerve.

thigh. In the gluteal region the fascia extends from the posterior belly of the gluteus maximus anteriorly to the tensor fascia femoris muscle. Between these two muscles the fascia is extremely thick as it overlies the gluteus medius and minimus. Thus, the tensor muscle is surrounded by fascia. The maximus is covered anteriorly by the fascia lata component, and posteriorly by a thinner investing fascia that blends with the epimysium and sends septa into the muscle belly. The gluteus medius-minimus compartment is covered by the stout fascia lata anterolaterally, and the posterior margin is the iliac bone. The sciatic nerve, which lies between the gluteus maximus and the pelvis-external rotator complex, may be compromised with increased pressure in this area (Fig. 3–16).

CLINICAL CORRELATION

The muscles involved in this location act to both extend and abduct the associated hip. Buttock tenderness and tenseness is a finding with involvement of these compartments.

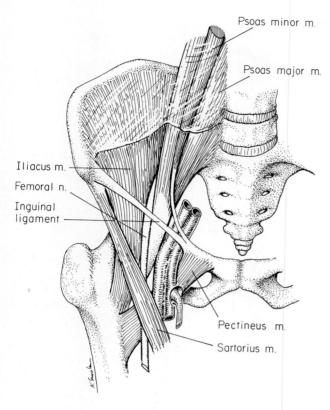

Psoas minor m.

Psoas major m.

Iliacus m.

Femoral n.

Inguinal
ligament

Pectineus m.

Sartorius m.

Figure 3–17   Iliacus compartment: anterior view of right hip and
pelvis.

Gluteal stretch pain with hip adduction or flexion could also reflect an underlying problem in the gluteal muscles. Paresthesias along the distal distribution of the sciatic nerve may also be present (Owen et al., 1978).

Iliacus Compartment

ANATOMY

The iliacus compartment is essentially very limited and consists primarily of the muscles of the inner wall of the pelvis — more specifically the psoas major, psoas minor, and iliacus (Fig. 3–17). Along with the femoral nerve, which travels through the pelvis in company with the psoas and iliacus muscles and then enters the leg through the inguinal canal adjacent to the rectus femoris, a relatively confined and functional compartment exists.

CLINICAL CORRELATION

Clinically this is a very rare location for a compartment syndrome to develop, although it has been described with hemorrhage in the pelvis and into the involved muscles (Goodfellow et al., 1967; Wells and Templeton, 1977). The classic presentation is seen in a patient who has hip flexion and pain with attempts at passive hip extension. Tenderness along the inguinal ligament may be noted, as well as dysesthesia around the knee and distally in the distribution of the saphenous nerve (the continuation of the femoral nerve) (Fig. 3–18). A clinical awareness of the possibility of a compartment syndrome occurring in this muscle group is important, as pressure measurements may be difficult to obtain.

Thigh: Anterior Compartment

ANATOMY

The fascia lata encircles the thigh. Medial and lateral intermuscular septa, which run from the fascia lata to the linea aspera along the posterior margin of the femur, help to compartmentalize the thigh muscles and divide the thigh into anterior and posterior groups. Laterally, the fascia is thicker as it is reinforced by tendinous fibers from the tensor fascia femoris and gluteus maximus, and in this location becomes the iliotibial tract.

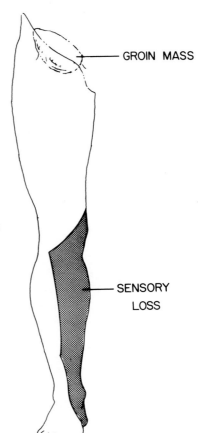

Figure 3–18   Clinical findings of an iliacus compartment syndrome.

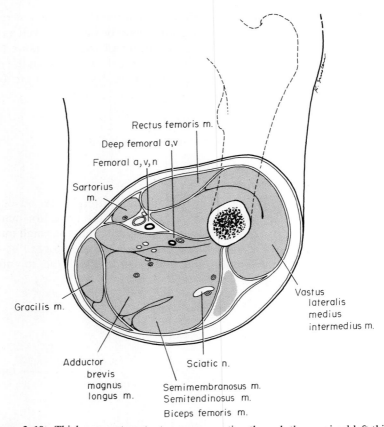

Rectus femoris m.

Deep femoral a,v

Femoral a,v,n

Sartorius
m.

Gracilis m.

Vastus
lateralis
medius
intermedius m.

Adductor
brevis
magnus
longus m.

Sciatic n.

Semimembranosus m.
Semitendinosus m.

Biceps femoris m.

Figure 3–19   Thigh compartments: transverse section through the proximal left thigh.

The muscles of the anterior compartment consist primarily of the quadriceps group. The sartorius muscle runs its course from the anterior superior iliac spine to the tibia anterior to the medial intermuscular septum, and therefore is located within the confines of the anterior compartment. All the muscles in this compartment are innervated by the femoral nerve, which also courses through this part of the thigh (Fig. 3–19).

The sensory component of the femoral nerve courses through the compartment in the adductor canal under cover of the sartorius. It terminates as the saphenous nerve, and supplies sensation to the medial leg and foot. The femoral artery runs with the nerve in the adductor canal. The artery exits the compartment distally in the thigh and becomes the popliteal artery at the level of the adductor hiatus.

CLINICAL CORRELATION

Knee extension, the primary responsibility of the quadriceps muscle, is the function that would be most affected by a compartment syndrome involving the thigh anterior compartment. In an effort to decrease stretch of the quadriceps muscle, the patient would tend to maintain the knee in an extended posture. Active quadriceps contraction, however, would probably cause pain in the anterior thigh, and the strength would be weakened as compared with the opposite, uninvolved limb. Concomitantly, passive flexion of the knee would stretch the ischemic muscle and cause pain in the anterior thigh area. Paresthesia may be noted over the knee and medial aspect of the leg and foot — the topographic areas supplied by the saphenous nerve. Of course, tenseness and tenderness over the anterior portion of the thigh would also be characteristic findings, but might be difficult to detect if there were a significant amount of subcutaneous tissue overlying the compartment.

Thigh: Posterior Compartment

ANATOMY

Anteriorly this compartment is limited by the medial and lateral intermuscular septa and the femur. The remaining posterior boundary is the fascia lata (Fig. 3–19).

The contents of this compartment can be divided into two major components. The hamstrings or knee flexors (biceps femoris, semitendinosus, semimembranosus) make up the posterior muscle group, and a more medial group consists of the adductor muscles (adductors magnus, brevis, and longus). The adductors are innervated by the obturator nerve, and the hamstrings by the sciatic nerve. The sciatic nerve courses entirely through the posterior compartment on its way to the leg.

CLINICAL CORRELATION

Involvement of the hamstring muscles could lead to loss of ability to actively and fully flex the knee against gravity. Passive knee extension may also cause intense pain in the posterior aspect of the thigh. Owing to the size of the sciatic nerve, a minimally elevated intracompartmental pressure may not lead to any neurologic changes. However, with significant pressure elevation, both sensory and motor function distal to the posterior thigh compartment muscles may occur if the sciatic nerve is compromised and becomes ischemic.

Paresis of the adductor muscles may be difficult to detect clinically in the acute phase. Tenderness and tenseness along the medial aspect of the thigh is an early sign. Paresthesias or dysesthesias along the course of the obturator nerve, which would primarily involve the medial aspect of the leg to the knee, may also assist the diagnosis.

Leg: Anterior Compartment

ANATOMY

This compartment is bound anteriorly by the crural fascia, which encircles the entire leg (Figs. 3–20, 3–21). Laterally the anterior intermuscular septum, which is an

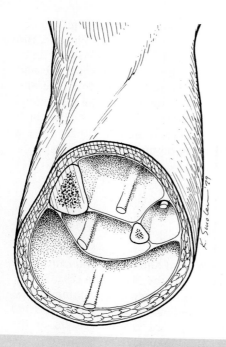

Figure 3–20   Four compartments of the leg.

LEG COMPARTMENTS

Anterior

TIBIALIS ANTERIOR m., EXTENSOR HALLUCIS LONGUS m., EXTENSOR DIGITORUM LONGUS m., and ANTERIOR TIBIAL a,v and n., PERONEUS TERTIUS m.

Lateral

PERONEUS LONGUS m., PERONEUS BREVIS m., and SUPERFICIAL PERONEAL n.

Deep posterior

TIBIALIS POSTERIOR m., FLEXOR DIGITORUM LONGUS m., FLEXOR HALLUCIS LONGUS m. and PERONEAL a. and v. and POSTERIOR TIBIAL a., v. and n.

Superficial posterior

SOLEUS m., PLANTARIS m., GASTROCNEMIUS m., and LESSER SAPHENOUS v. and PERONEAL COMMUNICATING n., (SURAL).

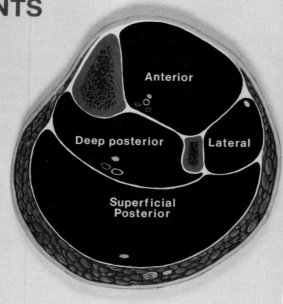

Figure 3–21   Leg compartments: transverse section through the middle portion of the left leg. (From Mubarak, S. J., and Hargens, A. R.: Diagnosis and management of compartment syndromes. *In* AAOS: Symposium on Injuries to the Leg. C. V. Mosby Co., St. Louis, 1980.)

extension of the crural fascia to the fibula, forms one boundary. Posteriorly the fibula, interosseous membrane, and tibia confine the muscles, nerves, and vessels within the anterior compartment.

The contents of the anterior compartment are primarily the muscles that dorsiflex the foot. These are the tibialis anterior, extensor digitorum longus, extensor hallucis longus, and, in the distal extent, the peroneus tertius. All muscles in this group are innervated by the deep peroneal nerve, which enters the compartment proximally around the fibular neck and exits distally as the anterior tibial nerve. This nerve supplies sensation to the first web space of the foot. The blood supply to this compartment consists of the anterior tibial artery, which continues in the foot as the dorsalis pedis artery (Fig. 3–22).

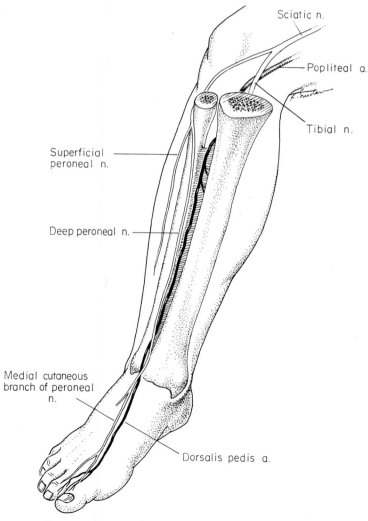

Figure 3–22 Anterior neurovascular structures of the leg.

CLINICAL CORRELATION

The anterior compartment of the leg is the most frequently involved location in the body for a compartment syndrome. Tenseness and tenderness lateral to the tibial crest is an important finding. Anterior leg pain associated with toe, foot, or ankle plantar flexion is characteristic. Sensory loss is confined to the first web space which, as noted, is the distribution of the deep peroneal nerve. Pain and limitation in active foot and toe dorsiflexion is another significant finding. The dorsalis pedis pulse is almost uniformly present (except when compartmental pressures exceed systolic pressures). Similarly, capillary refill is usually normal.

Leg: Lateral Compartment

ANATOMY

The limits of this compartment are anteriorly and laterally the crural fascia, medially the fibula and the anterior intermuscular septum, and posteriorly the posterior intermuscular septum (Figs. 3–20, 3–21). In a normal leg the anterior intermuscular septum can be found approximately halfway between the tibial crest and fibula.

The two muscles that make up the lateral compartment are the peroneus longus and brevis. These muscles are innervated by the superficial peroneal nerve, which is the major nerve in this compartment. The superficial peroneal nerve frequently exits through the crural fascia in the distal third of the leg, and divides at that stage into the dorsal medial cutaneous and dorsal intermediate cutaneous nerves of the foot. This division, however, in some cases may occur before the nerves traverse the fascia (Fig. 3–23).

Proximally, on its course around the fibular head to the anterior compartment, the deep peroneal nerve lies within the lateral compartment. Therefore, both the deep and superficial peroneal nerves are located within this compartment. No major vessel courses through it. The peroneal and anterior tibial arteries contribute to the blood supply of the peroneal muscles.

CLINICAL CORRELATION

The peroneal muscles act to evert the foot and ankle. Any weakness in this function, or pain in the lateral portion of the leg with active foot eversion or passive inversion, could indicate a compartment syndrome of the lateral compartment of the leg. A sensory deficit over the dorsum of the foot, perhaps not affecting the lateral border (sural nerve), is consistent with superficial peroneal nerve involvement (Fig. 3–24). Loss of sensation in the first web space, though not characteristic, may also occur if the deep peroneal nerve is compromised in its proximal course through the lateral compartment. Anatomically the superficial peroneal nerve in the distal half of the lateral compartment lies adjacent to the anterior intermuscular septum. Surgical

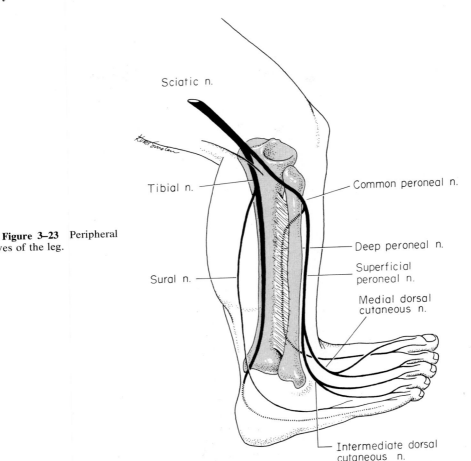

Sciatic n.

Tibial n.

Common peroneal n.

Figure 3–23 Peripheral
nerves of the leg.

Deep peroneal n.

Superficial
peroneal n.

Medial dorsal
cutaneous n.

Sural n.

Intermediate dorsal
cutaneous n.

awareness of this proximity is important, especially when distortion occurs in
normal anatomy as a result of alterations in compartmental pressures.

Leg: Superficial Posterior Compartment

ANATOMY

The muscles in this group are limited to the gastrocnemius, soleus, and plantaris
longus (Figs. 3–20, 3–21). Branches of the tibial nerve, posterior tibial artery, and
peroneal artery supply the muscles of this group. The main neurovascular structures
themselves, however, are located in the deep posterior compartment. The sural
nerve, which supplies sensation to the dorsal lateral portion of the ankle and foot, is
located in the posterior or superficial aspect of this compartment and is the only
significantly-sized nerve found here. This nerve frequently enters the subcutaneous
tissue of the leg in the proximal half of the calf.

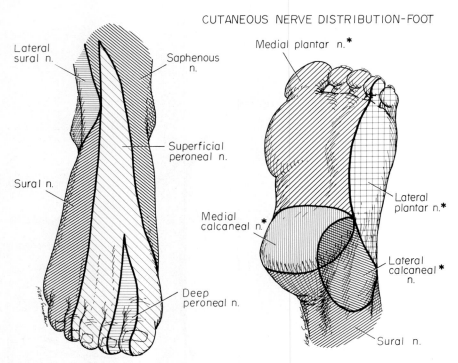

Figure 3–24   Distribution of the cutaneous nerves to the foot. * = Branches of the tibial nerve.

The compartment is entirely enveloped by fascia — posteriorly by the crural fascia and anteriorly by a thick, transverse, intermuscular septum. Medially, both fascial layers merge and unite at the tibia.

CLINICAL CORRELATION

The gastroc-soleus muscle complex is the major plantar flexor of the ankle. It is one of the strongest muscle groups of the body, and any minor paresis may be difficult to detect. However, posterior calf pain with active plantar flexion may be noted, as well as a similar pain occurring during passive ankle dorsiflexion. The sural nerve supplies sensation to the lateral aspect of the foot, and therefore a diminished sensory response in this location may occur with superficial posterior compartment pressure elevations.

Leg: Deep Posterior Compartment

ANATOMY

The transverse intermuscular septum posteriorly and the tibia, interosseous membrane, and fibula anteriorly envelop this compartment. Proximally the entire compartment is covered by the superficial posterior group of leg muscles (Fig. 3–25).

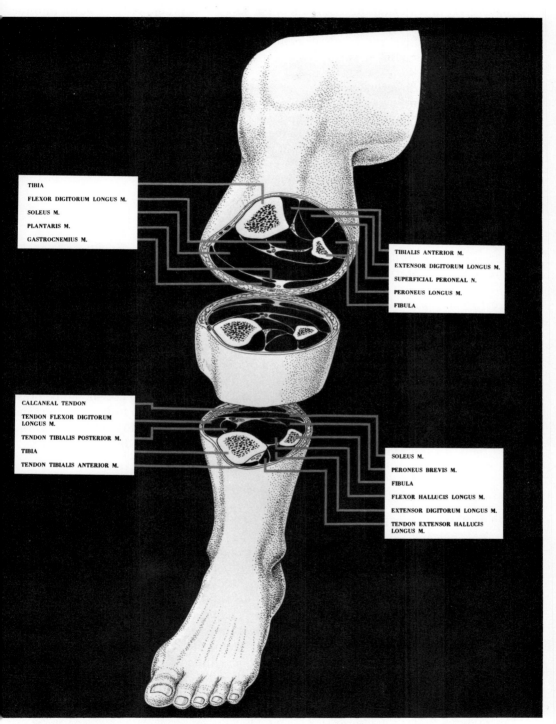

TIBIA

FLEXOR DIGITORUM LONGUS M.

SOLEUS M.

PLANTARIS M.

GASTROCNEMIUS M.

TIBIALIS ANTERIOR M.

EXTENSOR DIGITORUM LONGUS M.

SUPERFICIAL PERONEAL N.

PERONEUS LONGUS M.

FIBULA

CALCANEAL TENDON

TENDON FLEXOR DIGITORUM LONGUS M.

TENDON TIBIALIS POSTERIOR M.

TIBIA

TENDON TIBIALIS ANTERIOR M.

SOLEUS M.

PERONEUS BREVIS M.

FIBULA

FLEXOR HALLUCIS LONGUS M.

EXTENSOR DIGITORUM LONGUS M.

TENDON EXTENSOR HALLUCIS LONGUS M.

Figure 3–25   Leg compartments: transverse sections through the left leg at various levels. (From Mubarak, S. J., and Hargens, A. R.: Diagnosis and management of compartment syndromes. *In* AAOS: Symposium on Injuries to the Leg. C. V. Mosby Co., St. Louis, 1980.)

However, in the distal third of the leg, the superficial group narrows down into the Achilles tendon, and therefore in this area the fascia investing the deep compartment becomes superficial medially (adjacent to the tibia). In this location the transverse intermuscular septum is usually indistinct as it joins the crural fascia to attach firmly to the tibia.

The muscles in this group are the posterior tibialis, flexor hallucis longus, and flexor digitorum longus. The muscles are innervated by the tibial nerve and are vascularized by branches from either the posterior tibial or the peroneal arteries. The tibial nerve and artery lie adjacent to the posterior tibialis muscle, and course within this compartment. In the distal third of the leg, where the fascia of the deep compartment becomes superficial, the saphenous nerve and vein run along the fascia but not within the confines of the compartment.

CLINICAL CORRELATION

Tenseness of the deep posterior compartment is extremely difficult to detect, as the compartment itself is deep to the gastrocnemius and soleus muscles. Palpation of the muscles in this compartment is accomplished at the distal medial aspect of the tibia where the gastroc-soleus forms the Achilles tendon. With a compartment syndrome, passive stretch pain may be noted in the posterior deep compartment by dorsiflexing the toes or foot, as well as by everting the foot, and thus stretching the posterior tibialis muscle. Paresis in the toe flexors and possibly in the foot invertors may also be noted. Diminished sensation on the plantar aspect of the foot would be consistent with involvement of the posterior tibial nerve. As with the dorsalis pedis artery in the anterior compartment, the posterior tibial arterial pulse should be present and full in most cases of a deep posterior compartment syndrome. The surgical approach to the deep posterior compartment should take into consideration the proximity of the saphenous nerve and vein in the distal aspect of the leg.

Foot Compartments

ANATOMY

The foot is divided into four compartments, similar to those described in the hand. All are separated by fascia of varying thicknesses. The most superficial and strongest fascia is the plantar aponeurosis. Medial and lateral intermuscular septa extend dorsally from the plantar fascia to divide the foot into *medial, lateral,* and *central compartments.* The fourth, or *interosseous, compartment* lies dorsal to the above three, and is separated from them by a transverse fascial septum (Fig. 3–26).

The lateral compartment contains the flexor and abductor digit minimi. The medial compartment is of variable size and descriptions, but includes primarily the intrinsic muscles of the great toe, except for the adductor hallucis. The central space holds the adductor hallucis, quadratus plantae, and tendons of the flexor digitorum longus, flexor hallucis longus, and flexor digitorum brevis. The most dorsal compartment in the foot is the interosseous, containing the interosseous muscles to the toes. The plantar arches and digital nerves are located deep within the interosseous compartment.

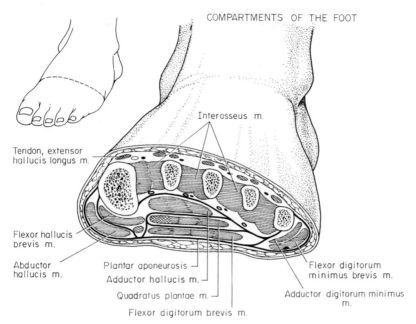

COMPARTMENTS OF THE FOOT

Interosseus m.

Tendon, extensor hallucis longus m.

Flexor hallucis brevis m.

Abductor hallucis m.

Plantar aponeurosis

Adductor hallucis m.

Quadratus plantae m.

Flexor digitorum brevis m.

Flexor digitorum minimus brevis m.

Adductor digitorum minimus m.

Figure 3–26

CLINICAL CORRELATION

Because most individuals have not developed fine motor skills of the feet, clinical separation of the various compartments of the foot is difficult to make. In general, tenseness and swelling of the foot should indicate the possibility of an underlying compartment syndrome. Limitations in specific foot or toe motions, however, may not be as easily detectable as in the hand, but attempts should be made to evaluate sensation of the toes as well as motion and pain elicited by passive stretch. One also, of course, must consider any previous loss of sensation due to other illnesses or pre-existing conditions. Similarly, claw toes or hammering of the toes may imply intrinsic muscle involvement, but may also have been present prior to the injury. Passive stretch pain and swelling may be the most useful signs in the evaluation of an acute foot compartment syndrome.

REFERENCES

Basmajian, J. V.: Muscles Alive: Their Functions Revealed by Electromyography, 2nd ed. Williams & Wilkins Co., Baltimore, 1967.

Blomfield, L. B.: Intramuscular vascular pattern in man. Proc. R. Soc. Med. 38:617, 1945.

Bourne, G. H.: Structure and Function of Muscle. Academic Press, New York, 1960.

Clark, W. E. LeG., and Blomfield, L. B.: The efficiency of intramuscular anastomoses, with observations on the regeneration of devascularized muscle. J. Anat. 79:15, 1945.

Edwards, D. A. W.: The blood supply and lymphatic drainage of tendons. J. Anat. 80:147, 1946.

Garfin, S. R., Tipton, C. M., Mubarak, S. J., Woo, S. L-Y., Hargens, A. R., and Akeson, W. H.: The role of fascia in the maintenance of muscle tension and pressure. J. Appl. Physiol., in press, 1981.

Gelberman, R. H., Zakaib, G. S., Mubarak, S. J., Hargens, A. R., and Akeson, W. H.: Decompression of
    forearm compartment syndromes. Clin. Orthop. 134:225–229, 1978.
Goodfellow, J., Fearn, C. R. D. A. and Matthews, J. M.: Iliacus haematoma. J. Bone Joint Surg. 49-B:
    748–756, 1967.
Hollinshead, W. H.: Textbook of Anatomy, 2nd ed. Harper & Row, New York, 1967.
Huber, G. C.: On the form and arrangement in fasciculi of striated voluntary muscle fibers. Anat. Rec.
    11:149, 1916.
Kanavel, A.: Infections of the Hand. Lea & Febiger, Philadelphia, 1933.
Owen, C. A., Woody, P. R., Mubarak, S. J., and Hargens, A. R.: Gluteal compartment syndromes. Clin.
    Orthop. 132:57–60, 1978.
Rydevik, B., and Lundborg, G.: Permeability of intraneural microvessels and perineurium following
    acute, graded experimental nerve compression. Scand. J. Plast. Reconstr. Surg. 11:179–187, 1977.
Saunders, R. L. de C. G., Lawrence, J., and Maciver, D. A.: Microradiographic studies of the vascular
    patterns in muscle and skin. In X-ray Microscopy and Microradiography. Academic Press, New
    York, 1957.
Sunderland, S.: Personal communication, 1978.
Wells, J., and Templeton, J.: Femoral neuropathy associated with anticoagulant therapy. Clin. Orthop.
    124:155–160, 1977.
Wollenberg, G. A.: Die Arterienversorgung von Muskelin und Sehner. Orthop. Clin. 14:312–331, 1905.

Chapter Four

PATHOPHYSIOLOGY
OF THE
COMPARTMENT
SYNDROME

Alan R. Hargens, Ph.D.,
and Wayne H. Akeson, M.D.

INTRODUCTION

The definition of a compartment syndrome provided earlier (Chapter 1) emphasizes that high pressure within a confined tissue space reduces blood flow sufficiently to jeopardize viability of intracompartmental tissues. The crucial role of volume-pressure distortions and consequent interference with normal intracompartmental blood circulation, implicit in the term "tamponade," was not clearly recognized until recently. Indeed, Volkmann (1881), whose name is historically associated with the limb deformity resulting from intracompartmental necrosis, was unaware of the underlying pathogenesis and central role of tamponade in compartment syndromes.

Present knowledge indicates that elevation of tissue fluid pressure lowers capillary blood flow, and that a sufficiently long period of microcirculatory ischemia produces necrosis of intracompartmental tissues. Recent studies of capillary blood pressure (Hargens et al., 1978) and capillary blood flow (Reneman et al., 1980) indicate that muscle microcirculation is compromised at tissue pressures as low as 30 to 40 mm Hg. Although capillary perfusion is inadequate to meet the metabolic demands of intracompartmental tissues, central arterial blood flow is typically normal in compartment syndromes (Fig. 4–1). Circulation of blood is confined to collateral circulations and low-resistance pathways (arteriovenous anastomoses, skin, compartments without tamponade) in compartment syndromes.

Another important variable that dictates the extent of tissue injury is pressurization time. Rorabeck and Clarke (1978) found that muscle and nerve dysfunction is progressively more severe as intracompartmental tamponade continues for four-, eight- and 12-hour periods. At an intracompartmental pressure of 30 mm Hg, nerve conduction velocity is significantly blocked after six to eight hours (Hargens et al.,

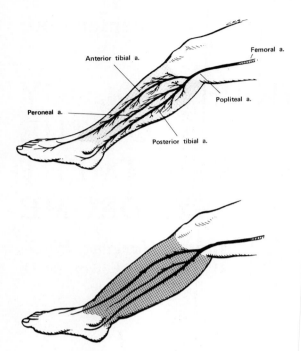

Anterior tibial a.

Femoral a.

Popliteal a.

Peroneal a.

Posterior tibial a.

Figure 4–1 Capillary blood ischemia associated with compartment syndromes. At tissue fluid pressures below 30 mm Hg, blood flows normally from arteries into arterioles and capillaries (upper leg). When pressure rises above 30 mm Hg, blood flow through intracompartmental capillaries is impeded while central artery and collateral circulations remain normal (lower leg). During capillary ischemia, blood flow is confined to large arteries, veins, and non-nutritional arteriovenous anastomoses. Typically, pulses are present in tissues distal to the region of elevated tissue pressure. This may give the physician a false sense of security in assuming that normal circulation is present in the muscle compartments.

1979). Quantitative measures of necrosis within entire muscles in dog hind limbs indicate that significant, irreversible injury is produced at 30 mm Hg after a pressurization period of eight hours (Hargens et al., 1981). However, long-term studies of muscle and nerve function are necessary to validate this conclusion directly.

The purpose of this chapter is to discuss: (1) the fluid accumulation within the compartment; (2) the relevance of several compartment syndrome models in animals; (3) the pressure-time thresholds that cause intracompartmental necrosis; and (4) the recommended pressure for decompression of impending compartment syndromes in clinical circumstances.

FLUID ACCUMULATION WITHIN COMPARTMENT

Historically, several mechanisms have been proposed to explain the pathogenesis of compartment syndromes: venous obstruction (Murphy, 1914; Brooks, 1922; Jepson, 1926); arterial occlusion (Harman and Guinn, 1948; Scully et al., 1961); arterial spasm (Griffiths, 1940; Eaton et al., 1965; Eaton and Green, 1972); and exertion (Vogt, 1943; Reneman, 1968). These theories have been replaced by one unified pathogenic factor for compartment syndromes (Matsen, 1975): elevated intracompartmental pressure, sufficiently high to compromise intracompartmental microcirculation.

The origin of the abnormally high intracompartmental pressure, however, is still somewhat obscure. Experimental and clinical studies of compartment syndrome pathophysiology (Hargens et al., 1977A,B, 1978; Mubarak et al., 1976, 1978A,B) indicate that intracompartmental fluid accumulation inside a tight, impermeable fascial enclosure is the initial, causative condition. For our animal studies we have used the anterolateral compartment of the dog (analogous to the separate anterior

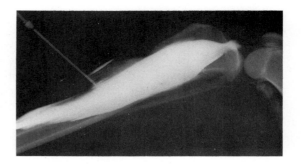

Figure 4-2 Lateral x-ray film of an anterolateral compartment in a canine hind limb, with contrast medium (Renografin 60) delineating the fascial boundaries. Muscles within this compartment are surrounded by a relatively noncompliant and fluid-impermeable fascia. (Reproduced with permission from Mubarak, S. J., et al.: The wick technique for measurement of intramuscular pressure: a new research and clinical tool. J. Bone Joint Surg. 58-A:1016–1020, 1976.)

and lateral compartments in humans) as our model. This compartment is a closed fluid container (Fig. 4–2). Little, if any, contrast media permeates the osseofascial connective tissue layer, and therefore hydrostatic pressure within one muscle compartment is not transmitted to adjacent compartments. Moreover, since tissue fluid pressure is equal throughout a given muscle compartment, fluids within a compartment are continuous (Mubarak et al., 1976).

Fluid accumulation originates from hemorrhage, extracellular edema, intracellular edema, or a combination of these mechanisms (Fig. 4–3). Hemorrhage can result from hematoma formation in hemophiliacs (Thomas, 1936), vessel lacerations (Horn and Sevitt, 1951), or fractures (Cohen, 1944; Eichler and Lipscomb, 1967; Grosz et al., 1973). Extracellular edema is produced by elevated capillary permeability following burns (Patman and Thompson, 1970), temporary ischemia (Whitesides et al., 1971), or increased capillary blood pressure (Reneman, 1968; Patman and Thompson, 1970). Intracellular edema results from postischemic swelling (Reneman, 1968; Patman and Thompson, 1970; Whitesides et al., 1971; Mubarak and Owen, 1975; Owen et al., 1979) associated with muscle membrane depolarization and intracellular water accumulation (Carrico et al., 1972; Shires et al., 1972; Arango et

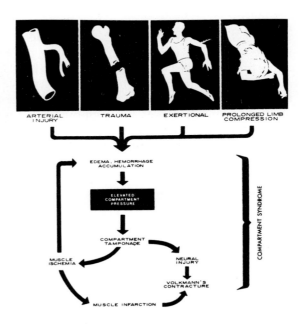

Figure 4-3 Pathophysiology of a compartment syndrome. A variety of conditions may initiate a sequence of events that produces a compartment syndrome. These conditions include arterial injury, trauma, exercise, or prolonged limb compression associated with alcohol or drug overdose. Common to all compartment syndromes is elevated intracompartmental pressure and subsequent ischemia. Without decompression, a self-perpetuating ischemia-edema process occurs, and irreversible damage, including Volkmann's contracture, may ensue. (Reproduced with permission from Mubarak, S. J., et al.: Muscle pressure measurement with the wick catheter. *In* Goldsmith, H. S. (ed.): Practice of Surgery. Harper & Row, Hagerstown, MD, 1978A, Chap. 20N, pp. 1–8.)

al., 1976). Shifts of water into muscle fibers probably result from high intracellular calcium concentrations following ischemia. Oberc and Engel (1977) detected abnormal accumulations of calcium in injured muscle by electron microscopy. Early findings demonstrate that extracellular calcium moves into the aqueous sarcoplasm of the muscle fibers. Later, calcium localizes in organelles, especially mitochondria and sarcoplasmic reticulum. Shen and Jennings (1972) observed calcium accumulation in mitochondria following acute ischemic injury in the myocardium.

Recent experimental findings in our laboratory suggest that intracellular swelling plays a major role in the generation of elevated intracompartmental pressure. Compartment syndromes are produced in canine anterolateral compartments after six hours of tourniquet ischemia in conjunction with partial arterial inflow of blood. After tourniquet removal, intracompartmental pressure, as measured by the wick catheter, often rises to 80 to 100 mm Hg. Perfusing the hind limb with 20 per cent mannitol via the femoral artery and vein produces a drop in intracompartmental pressure by as much as 80 mm Hg within one half-hour. Since mannitol almost completely permeates the capillary wall (Vargas and Johnson, 1977), this remarkable compartmental decompression suggests that most of the compartmental tamponade originates from intracellular swelling. It is known, for example, that mannitol and other hypertonic solutions (NaCl, inulin) withdraw intracellular water by osmosis (Vargas and Johnson, 1977). However, more studies are needed to validate these preliminary findings. Moreover, this evidence that postischemic swelling is probably related to intracellular edema does not lessen the important role of hemorrhage and extracellular edema as factors in the fluid accumulation of compartment syndromes.

COMPARTMENT SYNDROME INVESTIGATIONS

Tourniquet Ischemia

Postischemic swelling within muscle compartments is a typical response to tourniquet ischemia. Comprehensive studies by Whitesides and collaborators (Whitesides et al., 1971, 1980; Whitesides, 1978) examined alterations in enzymes, tissue pressure, muscle histology, and nerve function following several periods of tourniquet ischemia in the dog hind limb. Extensive edema, abnormal fluid sequestration, and tissue necrosis are produced by eight to ten hours of ischemia. Intracompartmental pressure rises upon tourniquet release. The magnitude of the pressure rise corresponds directly with the duration of tourniquet application. For example, in our studies, tissue pressure rises above arterial diastolic pressure in 50 per cent of hind limbs exposed to six-hour ischemic periods. Postischemic swelling in muscle compartments thus furthers the period of ischemia by elevating tissue pressure. Although the tourniquet is released and arterial inflow is resumed, capillary blood flow is occluded by the high tissue pressure.

Pneumatic tourniquet pressure and dog limb dimensions are important factors for reliable studies of limb ischemia (Whitesides, 1978). Tourniquet pressures of 400 to 600 mm Hg are necessary to elevate deep-tissue pressure sufficiently so that arterial inflow is totally obstructed. Tourniquet pressures of less than 400 mm Hg allow enough blood flow to accommodate the meager nutritional requirements of resting skeletal muscle (Whitesides, 1978). No edema is produced using tourniquet pressures of 400 to 600 mm Hg. On the other hand, at lower tourniquet pressures, venous obstruction occurs but some arterial flow persists. This produces considerable edema in the limb and should be avoided in order to obtain true ischemic conditions.

Light and electron microscopy reveal a great deal of variability of tissue damage, even among limbs exposed to identical periods of tourniquet ischemia (Whitesides, 1978). Muscle peripheries exhibit less necrosis than central portions. Edema is more pronounced in central regions also. Four-hour periods of ischemia produce no permanent damage in canine hind limbs. Six-hour episodes cause some injury of an irreversible type. Glycogen accumulation appears in electron micrographs after four- and six-hour ischemic periods, but is absent in eight-hour studies. Whitesides et al. (1971) conclude that the critical period of ischemia in dog muscle is six to eight hours.

Histochemical studies suggest that phosphorylase activity is significantly diminished in muscle exposed to four-hour periods of ischemia (Whitesides, 1978). At longer periods, phosphorylase activity is reduced proportionately. The disappearance of glycogen deposits after an eight-hour ischemia, however, suggests that other enzyme systems probably degrade the glycogen.

Recent studies of nerve function and muscle necrosis following four hours of tourniquet ischemia indicate that postischemic swelling and significant necrosis are produced in approximately 50 per cent of the experimental animals (Lee et al., 1981; Hargens et al., 1980). Peroneal nerve conduction is blocked just distal to the tourniquet after one half-hour in the canine hind limb. Failure of nerve conduction proceeds to more distal regions and finally occurs in the hind paw following one hour of tourniquet ischemia. During tourniquet application, intracompartmental pressure remains normal (4 ± 1 mm Hg), but postischemic tamponade occurs in approximately 50 per cent of the dogs (Table 4–1).

Significant muscle necrosis is associated with postischemic swelling in the compartment syndrome group of dogs. Uptake of technetium-99m pyrophosphate (99mTc-PYP) is a quantitative measure of total necrosis within the anterolateral compartment (Hargens et al., 1981). The ratio of 99mTc-PYP uptake in ischemic compartments to uptake in contralateral compartments of the compartment syndrome group is statistically higher (p < 0.05) than a comparable uptake ratio in dogs without compartment syndromes (Table 4–2). Qualitative histologic evaluations of muscle necrosis confirm these 99mTc-PYP findings.

Table 4–1 INTRACOMPARTMENTAL PRESSURE IN THE CANINE LIMB FOLLOWING FOUR HOURS OF TOURNIQUET APPLICATION*

	Compartment Syndrome Group (N = 5)	Noncompartment Syndrome Group (N = 7)
Control	4.4 ± 1.1	3.7 ± .95
After Tourniquet Removal:		
2 hours	40 ± 8.9	15 ± 2.9
24 hours	7.8 ± 1.9	6.7 ± 1.3
48 hours	7.8 ± 1.8	5.0 ± 1.2

*All values represent mean pressure ± S.E. within the anterolateral compartment.

Table 4–2 RATIO OF ^{99m}Tc-PYP IN POSTISCHEMIC COMPARTMENTS/
CONTRALATERAL COMPARTMENTS IN THE CANINE HIND LIMB
FOLLOWING FOUR HOURS OF TOURNIQUET APPLICATION*

	Compartment Syndrome Group (N = 5)	Noncompartment Syndrome Group (N = 7)
Uptake Ratio	14 ± 5.9	1.3 ± 1.7

*All values represent mean ratios ± S.E.

The different response of these two groups of dogs (compartment syndrome and noncompartment syndrome) may relate to the larger, less cylindric nature of hind limbs in the compartment syndrome group. Good tourniquet application is possible in long, thin canine hind limbs. Poor application is obtained in dogs with short, stubby hind limbs. Venous pressure slowly rises during tourniquet application in the compartment syndrome group, and thus partial arterial inflow, combined with venous congestion, probably contributes to compartment syndromes established in half of the hind limbs. This mechanism for producing a compartment syndrome is similar to that reported by Jepson (1926).

Compartment syndromes produced by tourniquet ischemia are highly variable in terms of the magnitude and duration of postischemic swelling. Moreover, owing to anatomic considerations, only 50 per cent of the experimental animals develop a compartment syndrome after four hours of tourniquet application (Lee et al., 1981). The advantage of a tourniquet model, however, lies in its duplication of intracompartmental tamponade by noninvasive procedures.

Inflated Balloon

Inflation of latex balloons within rabbit anterior compartments (Sheridan and Matsen, 1975) unfortunately has several deficiencies that reduce this model's relevance to compartment syndrome pathophysiology. First, insertion of the balloon is relatively invasive, and immunologic response to this foreign body is probable. Second, although intraballoon pressure is carefully controlled, intracompartmental tamponade is nonuniform; thus, intracompartmental pressure must be measured in several regions of the muscle in order to correlate necrosis quantitatively with tissue pressure. Third, insertion of the balloon probably alters the pressure-volume relations inherent within a muscle compartment with fully intact fascial boundaries. Finally, a note of caution regarding variability between species is necessary. Our studies of anterior compartments within rabbits indicate that this muscle group is not contained within a relatively closed osseofascial space, as are human anterior and canine anterolateral compartments (Hargens, unpublished observations).

Limb Compression

External compression models in rabbit hind limbs (Matsen et al., 1979) and human legs (Matsen et al., 1977) have provided valuable insights into tissue tolerance for increased pressure. Tibial nerve conduction is blocked completely in the rabbit hind limb at externally applied pressures of 60 to 80 mm Hg (Matsen et al., 1979). The time required to produce conduction block ranged between eight and 240 minutes in these authors' five-hour pressurization studies. In most animals, nerve conduction was blocked at an externally applied pressure of 80 mm Hg. However, tissue fluid pressure within a compartment was not measured. Furthermore, tissue fluid pressure is usually different from externally applied pressure, so that nerve tolerance to elevated tissue pressure was not known exactly. A model is needed in which the experimental compartment is easily accessible to physiologic studies during intracompartmental tamponade.

In another external compression model, Reneman and associates (1980, 1981) seal the rabbit hind paw in a pressurizable box and investigate venous pressure, intramuscular pressure, capillary blood flow, and arteriolar diameter. Arteriolar diameter increases when the gradient between arterial blood pressure and box pressure is lowered. A gradient of 24 mm Hg occludes muscle blood flow, whereas flow is renewed when the gradient reaches 31 mm Hg. The results suggest that, during compartment syndromes, muscle ischemia is produced by capillary occlusion rather than by venular collapse.

Studies in three normal individuals indicate some variability in motor and sensory nerve dysfunction related to elevated external pressure (Matsen et al., 1977). One subject, for example, tolerated only 55 mm Hg, whereas two others tolerated pressures of up to 65 and 75 mm Hg before sensory loss occurred. This variability in pressure-related disturbances was not attributable to individual differences in central blood pressure. However, more subjects at longer pressurization periods are needed, since Matsen and co-workers investigated only three normal males for periods of less than two hours. These pressurization times are considerably below those required for development of typical compartment syndromes in humans.

Other important studies by Matsen and associates in humans demonstrate that tolerance to elevated tissue pressure is reduced during limb elevation. For example, leg elevation to 52 cm above heart level reduced arterial blood pressure by 47 mm Hg in one subject and 43 mm Hg in another (Matsen et al., 1977). Compression of these elevated limbs by an airsplint indicates that nerve dysfunction occurs at a threshold pressure 35 mm Hg below the threshold level for a leg at heart level. Furthermore, intracompartmental pO_2 drops significantly upon leg elevation during external compression in normal subjects (Matsen et al., 1979). These findings are clinically important, and suggest that limb elevation in compartment syndromes and other conditions of decreased arterial perfusion is contraindicated.

Blood or Plasma Infusion

Infusion of autologous blood (Rorabeck and Clarke, 1978) or autologous plasma (Hargens et al., 1978, 1979) duplicates features relevant to the most common etiologies of compartment syndromes, namely, intracompartmental hemorrhage or edema caused by fracture, arterial injury, or high capillary permeability following compressive ischemia. Intracompartmental pressure is raised to any level by infusion of blood or plasma through a large needle into the compartment under study (Fig. 4–4). As previously demonstrated (Fig. 4–3), these infusion fluids are contained

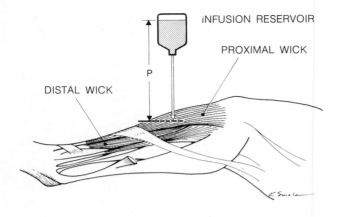

Figure 4–4 Pressure within the anterolateral compartment of the canine hind limb is raised by infusion of autologous blood or plasma. Intracompartmental pressure is recorded continuously by wick catheters. Pressure amplitude *(P)* is maintained by adjusting the height of the infusion reservoir, or alternatively by adjusting the rate of infusion through a pump apparatus. (Reproduced with permission from Hargens, A. R., et al.: Peripheral nerve-conduction block by high muscle-compartment pressure. J. Bone Joint Surg. 61-A:192–200, 1979.)

entirely within the relatively closed muscle compartment, although some resorption of infusate undoubtedly occurs in the lower range of intracompartmental tamponade. However, intracompartmental pressure is maintained at a constant, identical level throughout the muscle compartment for a desired period of time using this technique (Hargens et al., 1978). This compartment syndrome model offers the advantage of accessibility of involved muscles and reproducibility of intracompartmental tamponade, which are lacking in models described previously. However, one disadvantage is that all initial edema is extracellular in origin, and not intracellular as may occur after tourniquet ischemia. This model forms the basis for several studies of compartment syndrome pathophysiology and pressure-time thresholds of tissue necrosis that follow.

PRESSURE-TIME THRESHOLDS FOR INTRACOMPARTMENTAL NECROSIS

Volume-Pressure Relations in Muscle Compartments

In order to understand the relationships between tissue edema and intracompartmental tamponade, data on volume-pressure relations within skeletal muscle compartments are necessary. These data are obtained in the canine anterolateral compartment by stepwise, 1-ml injections of autologous plasma, with simultaneous measurements of increments in pressure. By this technique intracompartmental pressure is raised from a normal value of −4 mm Hg to levels of over 100 mm Hg. Results in eight dogs suggest the existence of a pressure range (−4 to 30 mm Hg) of relatively high tissue compliance followed by a pressure range (30 to 100 mm Hg) of relatively low tissue compliance (Fig. 4–5).

Our results regarding tissue compliance within the canine anterolateral compartment suggest that intracompartmental pressures above 30 mm Hg seriously jeopardize muscle viability. Above the threshold of 30 mm Hg, only small additions to intracompartmental edema volume elicit large increments in intracompartmental pressure, and vulnerability to ischemic necrosis rises proportionately. The notable drop in tissue compliance (slope of curve in Fig. 4–5) above 30 mm Hg probably represents a limit to which the surrounding fascial connective tissue is able to stretch.

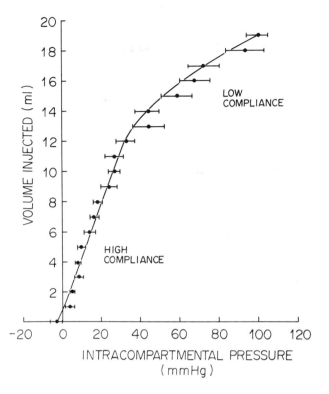

Figure 4–5 Volume-pressure relationships in anterolateral compartments of eight dogs. Tissue compliance is equal to the slope of plotted mean data (Δ volume/Δ pressure). Upon exceeding an intracompartmental pressure of 30 mm Hg, tissue compliance falls from 0.4 ml/mm Hg to 0.1 ml/mm Hg, and small additional edema volumes greatly raise intracompartmental pressure.

Intracompartmental pO_2

When intracompartmental pressure rises, there is a continuous reduction in tissue pO_2 and simultaneous rise in pCO_2 (Matsen et al., 1979; Hargens, unpublished observations). By increasing and decreasing intracompartmental pressure in the anterolateral compartment, barohysteresis of tissue pO_2 is observed (Fig. 4–6). This

Figure 4–6 Barohysteresis of pO_2 level in ten dogs occurs during compression and decompression of the canine anterolateral compartment. Thus, equilibrium pO_2 is higher in muscle during compression than tissue pO_2 during decompression of a muscle compartment. Importantly, the level of pO_2 is inversely proportional to muscle compartment pressure. Intracompartmental pressure is raised and lowered by adjusting height of the autologous plasma reservoir. (Reproduced with permission from Akeson, W. H., et al.: Muscle compartment syndromes and snake bites. *In* Hargens, A. R. (ed.): Tissue Fluid Pressure and Composition. Williams & Wilkins Co., Baltimore, 1981.)

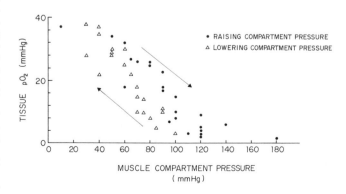

phenomenon is a retardation of the change in tissue pO_2 when intracompartmental pressure is changed. In other words, we have measured higher pO_2 during pressurization than during decompression, even though our oxygen microelectrode is allowed to reach equilibrium after each adjustment in intracompartmental pressure. Although pO_2 in canine muscle gradually drops below a normal level at intracompartmental pressures over 30 mm Hg, tissue necrosis cannot be inferred from these data alone. Whether determined by a mass spectrometer (Matsen et al., 1979) or miniature electrodes, tissue pO_2 measurements are insufficient in themselves to permit the seriousness of an impending compartment syndrome to be evaluated. Based on our measurement of pO_2 in canine muscle, and those of Matsen and associates (1979) in rabbit muscle, pO_2 is near zero mm Hg at intracompartmental pressures greater than 100 mm Hg. However, if this pressure is present for short periods (e.g., one hour), no tissue necrosis occurs. Thus, it is evident that the pressurization time factor is an important variable along with the amplitude of intracompartmental pressure.

Capillary Blood Pressure and Other Starling Forces

Since the pathophysiology of a compartment syndrome is related to abnormal fluid shifts between blood, extracellular space, and intracellular space, a detailed understanding of fluid balance within skeletal muscle is needed. Fluid transport across the capillary wall is determined by variables formulated by the Starling equation:

$$J_{tc} = L_p A \left[(P_c - P_t) - \sigma_p (\pi_c - \pi_t) \right]$$

where J_{tc} = net transcapillary fluid transport (ml/min)
  L_p = water conductivity (ml/min · mm^2 · mm Hg)
  A = capillary surface area (mm^2)
  P_c = capillary blood pressure (mm Hg)
  P_t = tissue fluid pressure (mm Hg)
  σ_p = capillary reflection coefficient (dimensionless, ranges between 0 and 1)
  π_c = capillary blood, protein osmotic pressure (mm Hg)
  π_t = tissue fluid, protein osmotic pressure (mm Hg)

Fluid is filtered out of the capillary ($J_{tc} > 0$) when $P_c - P_t > \sigma_p (\pi_c - \pi_t)$, usually at the arterial end of the capillary. Fluid is resorbed by the blood ($J_{tc} < 0$) when $P_c - P_t < \sigma_p (\pi_c - \pi_t)$, usually at the venous end of the capillary. When $P_c - P_t = \sigma_p (\pi_c - \pi_t)$, filtration exactly balances resorption of fluid across the capillary wall.

Capillary blood pressure, P_c, is determined by micropuncture using 1-μm pipeters connected to a servo-null micropressure device (Fig. 4–7). This technique allows direct, continuous recordings of blood pressure within arterioles, precapillary arterioles, true capillaries, postcapillary venules, and venules (Table 4–3). Capillary blood pressure, P_c, in canine muscle is normally 20 to 30 mm Hg. This range of pressure is nearly identical with that measured directly in nailfold capillaries of humans (Levick and Michel, 1978; Mahler et al., 1979).

Since capillary blood pressure normally ranges below 30 mm Hg, it is probable that tissue fluid pressures greater than this level reduce capillary perfusion through skeletal muscle. Blood flow is obstructed when tissue fluid pressure rises above intracapillary blood pressure, according to the "critical closing pressure" theory of Burton (1951) and Ashton (1962, 1975). Pressure in collapsible vessels such as veins

SERVO—NULL MICROPRESSURE SYSTEM

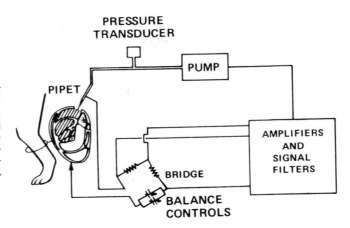

Figure 4–7 Measurement of capillary blood pressure in the canine anterolateral compartment, using the servo-null micropressure system. Surface microvasculature is exposed by an incision through skin and fascia. Micropuncture of muscle capillaries is accomplished with 1-μm pipets attached to a micromanipulator. Saline, warmed to 37 degrees C, suffuses the preparation continuously. Muscle microcirculation is visualized by microscope magnifications of 200×, using fiberoptic epilumination.

also rises as a consequence of elevated tissue fluid pressure (Ryder et al., 1944). However, postocclusive vasodilatation of smooth muscle in precapillary sphincters is highly unlikely in the presence of tissue fluid pressures over 30 mm Hg. In fact, elevation of venous pressure produces vasoconstriction (Burrows and Johnson, 1978). Under these conditions, capillary flow is probably shunted around capillary (nutritional) vessels and through arteriovenous anastomoses and other large blood vessels. These large, non-nutritional vessels represent a path of least resistance for blood flow, and readily explain the observation that distal pulses are present during compartment syndromes (see Fig. 4–1). This mechanism agrees with recent experimental evidence obtained by Reneman et al. (1980, 1981) in rabbit hind limbs.

Analysis of Starling pressures provides insights into the mechanism of postischemic swelling in skeletal muscle. Increased capillary permeability is a well known response to prolonged ischemia such as limb compression. Thus, osmotic forces in the Starling equation, which primarily resorb edema fluid in tissue, are probably inoperative. This condition leads to a point where tissue fluid pressure, P_t, is elevated to a level equal to capillary pressure, P_c. In cases in which arteriole or large artery injury occurs, P_t rises to a pressure equal to the blood pressure at the vessel's site of injury. Again, these circumstances elevate tissue fluid pressure sufficiently to occlude nutritional vessels and generate a compartment syndrome.

Table 4–3 MICROVASCULAR PRESSURE IN BLOOD VESSELS OF THE ANTEROLATERAL MUSCLE COMPARTMENT IN EIGHT DOGS

Vessel Type	Arteriole	Precapillary arteriole	True capillary	Postcapillary venule	Venule
Diameter Range (μm)	30–70	10–30	below 10	10–30	30–70
Range of Mean Pressure (mm Hg)	50–90	30–50	20–30	12–20	4–12

Blood Flow

Blood flow through skeletal muscle during intracompartmental tamponade is reduced. It is difficult to separate nutritional flow from non-nutritional flow, however, so the exact relationship between intracompartmental pressure and capillary blood flow is not known. At normal arterial pressure, an external pressure of 40 mm Hg is sufficient to decrease blood flow through a limb significantly (Ashton, 1966). Several investigators find a continuous decrease in muscle blood flow as tissue pressure rises (Dahn et al., 1967; Rorabeck and MacNab, 1975; Clayton et al., 1977; Sheridan et al., 1977; Rorabeck and Clarke, 1978; Matsen et al., 1979; Reneman et al., 1980, 1981). However, variations in capillary perfusion between one region and another in the same muscle compartment are probable, and this heterogeneity of blood flow may explain the patchy distribution of necrosis in compartment syndromes (Reneman, 1968; Hargens et al., 1981). These findings suggest that measurements of nutritional blood flow are needed to assess directly the relationship between elevated tissue pressure and reduced capillary perfusion within skeletal muscle. Labeled microspheres theoretically could provide this information.

Microscopy of Muscle and Nerve

The heterogeneity of capillary perfusion, discussed in the preceding section on muscle blood flow, manifests itself in a patchy distribution of muscle necrosis, especially at intracompartmental pressures of 30 to 40 mm Hg. Frozen biopsies of muscle obtained from the canine anterolateral compartment reveal a threshold level of necrosis at an intracompartmental pressure of 30 mm Hg after an eight-hour period of pressurization (Hargens et al., 1981). All muscle samples from compartments with normal pressure, 10 mm Hg for eight hours, and 20 mm Hg for eight hours, appear normal (Fig. 4–8).

Anterolateral compartments pressurized at 30 mm Hg and higher for eight hours incur progressively more severe and frequent muscle necrosis in direct proportion to the level of intracompartmental pressure. Degenerating fibers are present near fascicle peripheries at 30 mm Hg (Fig. 4–9). These peripheral fibers are destroyed by a connective tissue response. At 40 mm Hg cellular infiltration predominates (Fig. 4–10), whereas internal nuclei and split fibers are present in muscle samples from compartments pressurized at 60 mm Hg for eight hours (Fig. 4–11). Finally, uniform necrosis is evident throughout canine muscle pressurized at 120 mm Hg for eight hours (Fig. 4–12).

Light and electron-microscopic evaluations of peroneal nerve from pressurized and control muscle compartments support trends to greater necrosis at higher intracompartmental pressures (Hargens et al., 1979). For example, degeneration and swelling of axons as well as myelin disintegration occur in nerves pressurized above 50 mm Hg. These necrotic changes are distributed more uniformly at pressures of 100 and 120 mm Hg after eight hours. Swelling and degeneration of axonal contents are produced in unmyelinated axons also. It is difficult to establish a threshold level and duration of pressure for these degenerative histologic changes without quantitative and complete analysis of morphologic changes within the entire muscle and nerve. Therefore, we have borrowed the pyrophosphate-uptake technique from cardiac surgeons to quantitate irreversible necrosis of all tissues within an experimental muscle compartment.

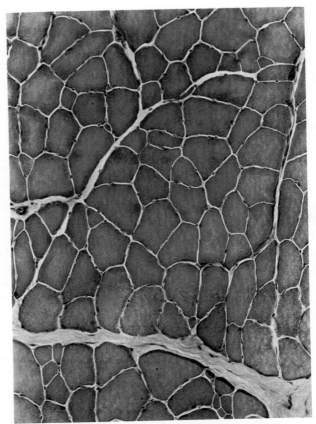

Figure 4–8 Normal structure is retained in canine muscle pressurized at 20 mm Hg for eight hours. Similarly, muscle pressurized at 10 mm Hg for eight hours and muscle from the contralateral control leg exhibit normal H & E staining and fiber architecture (100× original magnification, reproduced with permission from Hargens, A. R., et al.: Quantitation of skeletal-muscle necrosis in a model compartment syndrome. J. Bone Joint Surg.: 1981, in press.)

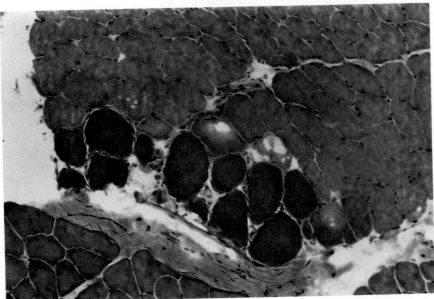

Figure 4–9 Representative muscle cross-section from a compartment pressurized at 30 mm Hg for eight hours. Patchy necrosis occurs as Fishback's degeneration, vacuolization, splitting, and hypertrophy of cells. Cellular infiltration occurs primarily along connective tissue planes (100× original magnification, reproduced with permission from Hargens, A. R., et al.: Quantitation of skeletal-muscle necrosis in a model compartment syndrome. J. Bone Joint Surg.: 1981, in press.)

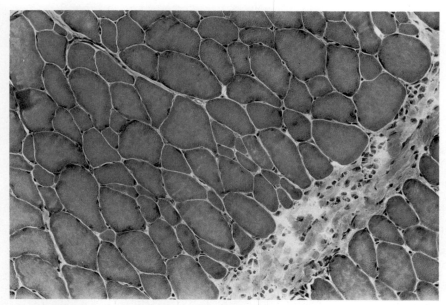

Figure 4–10   Fiber degeneration and cellular infiltration are more prevalent in muscle pressurized at 40 mm Hg for eight hours than at lower pressures (100× original magnification, reproduced with permission from Hargens, A. R., et al.: Quantitation of skeletal-muscle necrosis in a model compartment syndrome. J. Bone Joint Surg.: 1981, in press.)

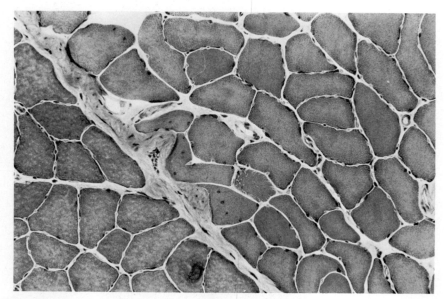

Figure 4–11   At 60 mm Hg (eight hours), internal nuclei and fiber splitting occur in addition to the degenerative processes evident at lower pressures (100× original magnification, reproduced with permission from Hargens, A. R., et al.: Quantitation of skeletal-muscle necrosis in a model compartment syndrome. J. Bone Joint Surg.: 1981, in press.)

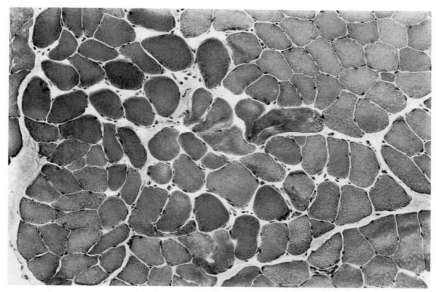

Figure 4–12 Representative cross-section of canine muscle after an eight-hour pressurization at 120 mm Hg. Cellular infiltration and fiber degeneration occur uniformly throughout the entire cross-section (100× original magnification, reproduced with permission from Hargens, A. R., et al.: Quantitation of skeletal-muscle necrosis in a model compartment syndrome. J. Bone Joint Surg.: 1981, in press.)

Uptake of Pyrophosphate

Irreversible muscle necrosis in cardiac muscle is presently identified and quantitated by measurement of technetium-99m stannous pyrophosphate (^{99m}Tc-PYP) uptake (Lewis et al., 1977; Reimer et al., 1977). In a series of 39 dogs we injected ^{99m}Tc-PYP intravenously, and measured uptake in canine muscle pressurized at levels of from 0 to 120 mm Hg for eight hours. Uptake in each experimental compartment was compared with that in the contralateral, control compartment of each dog. Thus, ^{99m}Tc-PYP uptake was expressed as a ratio (pressurized muscle uptake/control muscle uptake). Six dogs were studied at each pressure level. The threshold pressure and time for muscle necrosis was 30 mm Hg applied for eight hours. Significantly higher uptake of ^{99m}Tc-PYP ($p < 0.05$) was present at this level and duration of compartmental tamponade. The amount of necrosis increased in a near-exponential manner above this threshold pressure of 30 mm Hg (Fig. 4–13).

This pressure-time threshold (30 mm Hg for an eight-hour period) for muscle necrosis at normal blood pressure is significantly reduced under conditions of hemorrhagic hypotension (Zweifach et al., 1980). In this study, pressure was lowered from 107 ± 10 mm Hg to 65 mm Hg in six dogs within a period of 45 minutes. The left anterolateral compartment was pressurized to 20 mm Hg for six hours, while the contralateral compartment served as a control. After six hours' pressurization, the blood was returned to the animal. Matsen and collaborators (1980B) found decreased nerve function associated with hemorrhagic hypotension and relative low-pressure compartment syndromes. Our pyrophosphate uptake data were expressed as a ratio

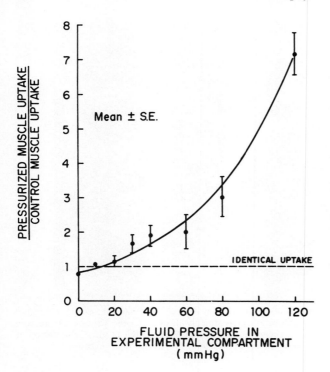

Figure 4–13 Ratio of ^{99m}Tc-PYP uptake in pressurized muscle/contralateral control muscle in 38 dogs. Significantly greater uptake occurs at an intracompartmental pressure threshold of 30 mm Hg. All pressurization times are eight hours. Each mean ± S.E. represents six dogs. (Reproduced with permission from Hargens, A. R., et al.: Quantitation of skeletal-muscle necrosis in a model compartment syndrome. J. Bone Joint Surg.: 1981, in press.)

Figure 4–14 Compared to muscle compartments with normal blood pressure perfusion (curve plotted from uptake ratios, •), compartments pressurized at 20 mm Hg in hypotensive dogs have a lower threshold for ischemic necrosis (▲ data point). Each mean ± S.E. represents the ratio of ^{99m}Tc-PYP uptake in pressurized muscle/control muscle in six dogs. Necrosis in compartments pressurized at 20 mm Hg for six hours in hypotensive dogs corresponds to the same amount of necrosis produced at 45–50 mm Hg for eight hours in dogs with normal blood pressure. (Reproduced with permission from Zweifach, S. S., et al.: Skeletal muscle necrosis in pressurized compartments associated with hemorrhagic hypotension. J. Trauma 20:941–947, 1980.)

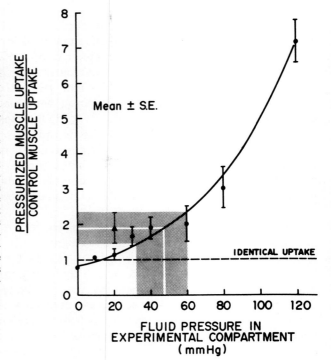

(pressurized muscle uptake/control muscle uptake). In these shock experiments, significant uptake (p<0.05) was present in compartments pressurized for six hours at 20 mm Hg (Fig. 4–14). In fact, our data suggest that 20 mm Hg for six hours produces the same amount of muscle necrosis as 40 to 50 mm Hg for eight hours under conditions of normal blood pressure.

Since trauma and hemorrhagic hypotension are often associated with acute compartment syndromes, these results are particularly relevant to the clinical diagnosis of an impending compartment syndrome. Certainly our hypotensive state of 65 mm Hg is within a blood pressure range confronted in clinical cases of shock. These findings indicate that ischemic necrosis occurs in a hypotensive patient at intracompartmental pressure considerably below the threshold level in those with normal blood pressure.

Nerve Function

Intracompartmental nerve dysfunction also occurs at a pressure threshold level of 30 to 40 mm Hg. Nerve conduction velocity and action potential amplitude were evaluated by electromyography at normal and elevated compartment pressures in the dog hind limb (Fig. 4–15). Under conditions of elevated intracompartmental pressure, action potential amplitude diminished, and subsequently failed completely. The period of pressurization required for nerve failure was directly proportional to intracompartmental pressure. At pressures between 100 to 120 mm Hg, conduction was blocked completely after 30 to 60 minutes (Fig. 4–16). Complete failure of

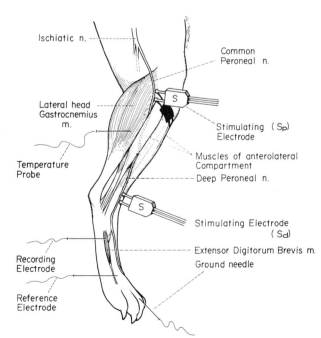

Figure 4–15 Deep peroneal nerve function is evaluated by measuring conduction velocity between proximal and distal stimulation points Sp and Sd and action potential amplitude in the extensor digitorum brevis muscle. Limb temperature is held constant at 36 degrees C. (Reproduced with permission from Hargens, A. R., et al.: Peripheral nerve-conduction block by high muscle-compartment pressure. J. Bone Joint Surg. 61-A:192–200, 1979.)

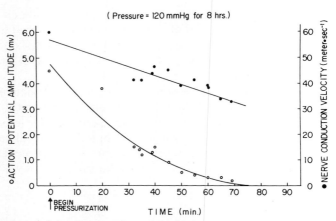

Figure 4–16   Sequential action potential amplitudes (○ data) and conduction velocities (● data) in an anterolateral compartment pressurized at 120 mm Hg. Nerve function is progressively lost, with large, faster-conducting neurons preferentially blocked. (Reproduced with permission from Hargens, A. R., et al.: Peripheral nerve-conduction block by high muscle-compartment pressure. J. Bone Joint Surg. 61-A:192–200, 1979.)

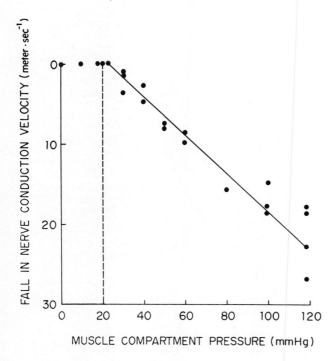

Figure 4–17   Fall in nerve conduction velocity is greater at higher intracompartmental pressures. Conduction velocity is reduced significantly at a threshold level of 30 mm Hg after six to eight hours. The fall in conduction velocity as a function of intracompartmental pressure suggests that faster-conducting fibers are more susceptible to ischemic injury than slower-conducting fibers. Conduction velocity remains normal at intracompartmental pressures of 0, 10, and 20 mm Hg. Each point represents one animal. (Reproduced with permission from Hargens, A. R., et al.: Peripheral nerve-conduction block by high muscle-compartment pressure. J. Bone Joint Surg. 61-A:192–200, 1979.)

conduction was never produced at pressures lower than 50 mm Hg. Importantly, however, partial conduction impairment occurred after six to eight hours of pressurization at 30 mm Hg (Fig. 4–17). These findings suggest that large, faster-conducting motor neurons are more susceptible to ischemic failure than small, slower-conducting neurons (Hargens et al., 1979).

These results support the thorough study of Rorabeck and Clarke (1978), which demonstrates that peroneal nerve conduction is partially blocked after 2½ hours at 40 mm Hg. The compartment syndrome produced by these authors is generated by autologous blood infusion into the canine anterolateral compartment, a model similar in many respects to our infusion of autologous plasma. Conduction velocity returns to near-normal in a compartment pressurized as high as 160 mm Hg if fasciotomy is performed within four hours (Rorabeck and Clarke, 1978). It is important to note, however, that these experiments indicate that conduction velocity remains abnormal at a pressure of 40 mm Hg if the compartment is not decompressed within 12 hours. Thus, the weight of several lines of evidence suggests that significant, irreversible damage to nervous tissues is produced at intracompartmental pressures between 30 and 40 mm Hg after six to 12 hours.

In order to distinguish mechanical compression nerve dysfunction from ischemic nerve dysfunction, we tested two groups of dogs (Mubarak et al., 1979). In the pressurized group, autologous plasma was infused intramuscularly to elevate the pressure within the anterolateral muscle compartment. The infusion pressure in the compartment was monitored with proximally and distally placed wick catheters. Within one to two minutes the pressure was elevated to greater than 100 mm Hg (100 to 120). Peroneal nerve conduction studies were repeated immediately after obtaining the desired pressure, and at ten-minute or shorter intervals throughout the experiment. The exact time of conduction loss proximal and distal to the compartment was recorded. In the ischemic group of nine dogs, after the baseline nerve conduction data had been obtained, intravenous air embolism was utilized to cause sudden death of the animal. Cardiorespiratory function ceased in 30 seconds in all cases. Conduction studies were performed at the same intervals as for the pressurized group.

In the pressurized dogs, peroneal nerve conduction was blocked at 58 ± 7 minutes upon stimulation at a site proximal to the anterolateral compartment. On the other hand, conduction failure occurred after only 30 ± 2 minutes upon proximal stimulation in the ischemic group. In the compartment syndrome model the distal site of peroneal nerve stimulation never diminished, owing to adequate collateral circulation via the posterior compartment. In the pressurized group the nerve loss appeared to be due to ischemia alone. Although the delay in nerve conduction differed in this group from that in the ischemic group, the ischemia in the compartment was probably less complete when pressurized to only 100 mm Hg than in the sacrificed animals. Furthermore, the location of the ischemia in the pressurized animals occurred between the proximal and distal nerve stimulation sites. Thus one would expect that the time for nerve conduction failure in this area must be more than 30 minutes but less than 62 minutes. If pressure is an additive factor to ischemia, one would expect that the time until loss of nerve function would be faster (less than 30 minutes). These studies suggest that, in compartment syndromes, neurologic loss is due to an elevated tissue fluid pressure occluding the nerve microcirculation, and thus causing ischemic failure of nerve conduction.

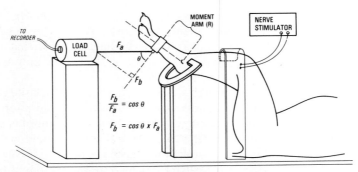

Figure 4–18   Chronic-boot apparatus for testing long-term muscle function in the canine anterolateral compartment. Anterolateral muscles are stimulated by percutaneous electrodes placed over the peroneal nerve. Muscle-contraction force F_b is calculated from force F_a, recorded by a load cell. Torque equals $F_b \times R$.

Muscle Function

Less information is available on threshold pressure and time parameters that produce muscle dysfunction. Only qualitative data exist in short-term studies using an inflatable balloon model (Sheridan et al., 1977), which has only limited relevance to physiologic compartment syndromes. No long-term study of muscle function after varying pressure levels and times is presently available.

It is necessary to develop a reliable technique for long-term evaluation of muscle function after a compartment syndrome or ischemic insult, in order to quantify reversible and irreversible changes in muscle performance following experimental compartment syndromes. A boot apparatus, recently designed in our laboratory, meets most criteria required for long-term studies of function in the canine anterolateral compartment (Fig. 4–18).

RECOMMENDED PRESSURES FOR COMPARTMENT DECOMPRESSION

At present opinions differ with respect to a threshold pressure at which fasciotomy is required to decompress a threatened compartment syndrome (Table 4–4). Although injection and infusion techniques measure pressures that are systematically higher than pressures measured by the wick technique, larger differences of opinion regarding a threshold pressure for fasciotomy are not explained by methodologic peculiarities alone. Although there is a broad spectrum of pressure-time thresholds among patients with threatened compartment syndromes, we believe that the severe sequelae of an untreated compartment outweigh the disadvantages of performing fasciotomies on the few patients whose pressures are greater than 30 mm Hg and who may never develop a Volkmann's contracture. Definitive answers to questions of long-term viability of skeletal muscle and nerve, however, await quantitative studies of muscle and nerve function over a period of several months following compartmental pressurization.

Table 4–4 RECOMMENDED PRESSURES FOR COMPARTMENT DECOMPRESSION

Investigators	Pressure Threshold	Technique	Experimental Indication
	NORMAL BLOOD PRESSURE		
Akeson et al., 1980	30 mm Hg after 8 hours	Wick	Animal and patient studies
Ashton, 1962	30 mm Hg	Air splint	50% reduction in blood flow
Halpern and Nagel, 1979	40 mm Hg	Needle injection	Clinical evaluation
Hargens et al., 1978	30 mm Hg	Wick	Fluid balance in dogs
Hargens et al., 1979	30 mm Hg after 6–8 hours	Wick	Nerve dysfunction in dogs
Hargens et al., 1981	30 mm Hg after 8 hours	Wick	Irreversible muscle necrosis in dogs
Matsen et al., 1976	40 mm Hg	Needle infusion	Rabbit studies
Matsen, 1978	65 mm Hg	Needle infusion	Laboratory and clinical experience
Matsen et al., 1980A	55 mm Hg	Needle infusion	Patient experience
Mubarak et al., 1976	30 mm Hg	Wick	Animal studies and clinical experience
Mubarak et al., 1978A, B	30 mm Hg	Wick	Clinical experience
Owen et al., 1979	30 mm Hg	Wick	Compartment syndromes due to limb compression
Rorabeck and Clarke, 1978	Below 40 mm Hg after 12 hours	Wick	Nerve dysfunction in dogs
Rorabeck, personal communication, 1980	30 mm Hg	Slit or wick catheter	Laboratory and clinical studies
Whitesides et al., 1975	50–70 mm Hg	Needle injection	Clinical experience
Whitesides et al., 1980	55–60 mm Hg	Needle injection	Clinical experience
	LOW BLOOD PRESSURE		
Matsen et al., 1980B	Below 40 mm Hg at mean blood pressure of 75 mm Hg	Needle infusion	Hemorrhaged rabbits
Zweifach et al., 1980	20 mm Hg after 6 hours at mean blood pressure of 65 mm Hg	Wick	Hemorrhaged dogs

SUMMARY

The pathogenesis of a compartment syndrome is primarily related to fluid or water accumulation in extracellular or intracellular spaces, respectively. Either of these two sites of accumulation increases intracompartmental volume, which in turn raises intracompartmental pressure as a consequence of low fascial compliance (Hargens et al., 1978). After reaching a threshold level of intracompartmental pressure, muscle ischemia is sufficient to produce irreversible myoneural necrosis after a threshold period of pressurization. Acute ischemia alone (e.g., limb compression) can elevate capillary permeability and produce interstitial edema. Subsequently, interstitial fluid pressure rises above a threshold level, and the vicious cycle of microvascular occlusion and ischemia ensues. In addition, a post-traumatic capillary or arteriolar fluid leak alone can raise interstitial fluid pressure to precipitate the ischemia-edema cycle, as just described. Thus, a multifactorial etiology is apparent for the pathogenesis of compartment syndromes in humans.

The weight of recent evidence indicates that significant intracompartmental necrosis is produced at a threshold-pressure level and duration of 30 mm Hg and eight hours. This pressure threshold is lowered under conditions of hemorrhagic hypotension. However, this tissue damage may represent injury that is reversible during subsequent myoneural regeneration. Only long-term tests of muscle and nerve function will provide objective criteria for defining a matrix of pressure-time variables that produce irreversible necrosis. Until these data are available and since time factors are usually unknown, we suggest that impending compartment syndromes require decompressive fasciotomy at an intracompartmental pressure of 30 mm Hg.

REFERENCES

Akeson, W. H., Hargens, A. R., Garfin, S. R., and Mubarak, S. J.: Muscle compartment syndromes and snake bites. *In* Hargens, A. R. (ed.): Tissue Fluid Pressure and Composition. Williams & Wilkins Co., Baltimore, 1981, pp. 215–226.

Arango, A., Illner, H., and Shires, G. T.: Roles of ischemia in the induction of changes in cell membrane during hemorrhagic shock. J. Surg. Res. 20:473–476, 1976.

Ashton, H.: Critical closing pressure in human peripheral vascular bed. Clin. Sci. 22:79–87, 1962.

Ashton, H.: Effect of inflatable plastic splints on blood flow. Br. Med. J. 2:1427–1430, 1966.

Ashton, H.: The effect of increased tissue pressure on blood flow. Clin. Orthop. 113:15–26, 1975.

Brooks, B.: Pathologic changes in muscle as a result of disturbances of circulation, an experimental study of Volkmann's ischemic paralysis. Arch. Surg. 5:188–216, 1922.

Burrows, M. E., and Johnson, P. C.: Effect of pressure variations on wall tension and volume flow in arterioles of cat mesentery. Fed. Proc. 37:874, 1978.

Burton, A. C.: On the physical equilibrium of small blood vessels. Am. J. Physiol. 164:319–329, 1951.

Carrico, C. J., Baker, C. R. F., Jr., Cunningham, J. N., and Shires, G. T.: The extracellular fluid and its measurement. *In* Malinin, T. I., Zeppa, R., Gollam, F., and Callahan, A. B. (eds.): Reversibility of Cellular Injury Due to Inadequate Perfusion. Charles C Thomas, Springfield, 1972, pp. 84–98.

Clayton, J. M., Hayes, A. C., and Barnes, R. W.: Tissue pressure and perfusion in the compartment syndrome. J. Surg. Res. 22:333–339, 1977.

Cohen, S. M.: Traumatic arterial spasm. Lancet 1:1–6, 1944.

Dahn, I., Lassen, N. A., and Westling, H.: Blood flow in human muscles during external pressure or venous stasis. Clin. Sci. 32:467–473, 1967.

Eaton, R. G., and Green, W. T.: Epimysiotomy and fasciotomy in the treatment of Volkmann's ischemic contracture. Orthop. Clin. North Am. 3:175–185, 1972.

Eaton, R. G., Green, W. T., and Stark, H. A.: Volkmann's ischemic contracture in children. J. Bone Joint Surg. 47-A:1289, 1965.

Eichler, G. R., and Lipscomb, P. R.: The changing treatment of Volkmann's ischemic contractures from 1955 to 1965 at the Mayo Clinic. Clin. Orthop. 50:215–223, 1967.

Griffiths, D. L.: Volkmann's ischaemic contracture. Br. J. Surg. 28:239–260, 1940.

Grosz, C. R., Shaftan, G. W., Kottmeier, P. K., and Herbsman, H.: Volkmann's contracture and femoral shaft fractures. J. Trauma 13:129–131, 1973.

Halpern, A. A., and Nagel, D. A.: Compartment syndromes of the forearm: early recognition using tissue pressure measurements. J. Hand Surg. 4:258–263, 1979.

Hargens, A. R., Akeson, W. H., Mubarak, S. J., Owen, C. A., Evans, K. L., Garetto, L. P., Gonsalves, M. R., and Schmidt, D. A.: Fluid balance within the canine anterolateral compartment and its relationship to compartment syndromes. J. Bone Joint Surg. 60-A:499–505, 1978.

Hargens, A. R., Akeson, W. H., Mubarak, S. J., Owen, C. A., and Garetto, L. P.: Tissue fluid states in compartment syndromes. *In* Lewis, D. H. (ed.): Recent Advances in Basic Microcirculatory Research, Part I. S. Karger, Basel, Bibliotheca Anatomica 15:108–111, 1977A.

Hargens, A. R., Gershuni, D. H., Gould, R. N., Zweifach, S. S., Mubarak, S. J., and Akeson, W. H.: Tissue necrosis associated with tourniquet ischemia. XI. European Conf. for Microcirc., Garmisch-Partenkirchen, Germany, Sept., 1980.

Hargens, A. R., Mubarak, S. J., Owen, C. A., Garetto, L. P., and Akeson, W. H.: Interstitial fluid pressure in muscle and compartment syndromes in man. Microvasc. Res. 14:1–10, 1977B.

Hargens, A. R., Romine, J. S., Sipe, J. C., Evans, K. L., Mubarak, S. J., and Akeson, W. H.: Peripheral nerve-conduction block by high muscle-compartment pressure. J. Bone Joint Surg. 61-A:192–200, 1979.

Hargens, A. R., Schmidt, D. A., Evans, K. L., Gonsalves, M. R., Garfin, S. R., Mubarak, S. J., Hagan, P. L., and Akeson, W. H.: Quantitation of skeletal-muscle necrosis in a model compartment syndrome. J. Bone Joint Surg., 1981, in press.

Harman, J. W., and Guinn, R. P.: The recovery of skeletal muscle fibers from acute ischemia as determined by histologic and chemical methods. Am. J. Pathol. 24:741–755, 1948.

Horn, J. S., and Sevitt, S.: Ischemic necrosis and regeneration of the tibialis anterior muscle after rupture of the popliteal artery. J. Bone Joint Surg. 33-B:348–359, 1951.

Jepson, P. N.: Ischemic contracture. Experimental study. Am. Surg. 84:785–795, 1926.

Lee, Y. F., Gould, R. N., Hargens, A. R., Mubarak, S. J., and Akeson, W. H.: The effects of tourniquet ischemia on nerve and skeletal muscle. Orthop. Trans. 5, 1981, in press.

Levick, J. R., and Michel, C. C.: The effects of position and skin temperature on the capillary pressures in the fingers and toes. J. Physiol. (Lond.) 274:97–109, 1978.

Lewis, M., Buja, L. M., Saffer, S., Michelevich, D., Stokely, E., Lewis, S., Parkey, R., Bonte, F., and Willerson, J.: Experimental infarct sizing using computer processing and a three-dimensional model. Science 197:167–169, 1977.

Mahler, F., Muheim, M. H., Intaglietta, M., Bollinger, A., and Anliker, M.: Blood pressure fluctuations in human nailfold capillaries. Am. J. Physiol. 236:H888–H893, 1979.

Matsen, F. A., III: Compartmental syndrome: a unified concept. Clin. Orthop. 113:8–14, 1975.

Matsen, F. A., III: Compartmental syndromes. Sound-slide program no. 702. Presented at the Annual Meeting, Am. Acad. Orthop. Surg., Dallas, TX, Feb. 25, 1978.

Matsen, F. A., III, King, R. V., Krugmire, R. B., Jr., Mowery, C. A., and Roche, T.: Physiological effects of increased tissue pressure. Int. Orthop. 3:237–244, 1979.

Matsen, F. A., III, Mayo, K. A., Krugmire, R. B., Jr., Sheridan, G. W., and Kraft, G. H.: A model compartment syndrome in man with particular reference to the quantification of nerve function. J. Bone Joint Surg. 59-A:648–653, 1977.

Matsen, F. A., III, Mayo, K. A., Sheridan, G. W., and Krugmire, R. B., Jr.: Monitoring of intramuscular pressure. Surgery 79:702–709, 1976.

Matsen, F. A., III, Winquist, R. A., and Krugmire, R. B., Jr.: Diagnosis and management of compartmental syndromes. J. Bone Joint Surg. 62-A:286–291, 1980A.

Matsen, F. A., III, Wyss, C. R., King, R. V., and Simmons, C. W.: Effect of acute hemorrhage on transcutaneous, subcutaneous, intramuscular, and arterial oxygen tensions. Pediatrics 65:881–883, 1980B.

Mubarak, S. J., Hargens, A. R., Garfin, S. R., Akeson, W. H., and Evans, K. L.: Loss of nerve function in compartment syndromes: pressure versus ischemia? Trans. Orthop. Res. Soc., 25th Ann. Meeting, San Francisco, CA, Feb. 20, 1979, p. 275.

Mubarak, S. J., Hargens, A. R., Owen, C. A., and Akeson, W. H.: Muscle pressure measurement with the wick catheter. In Goldsmith, H. S. (ed.): Practice of Surgery. Harper and Row, Hagerstown, MD, 1978A, Chap. 20N, pp. 1–8.

Mubarak, S. J., Hargens, A. R., Owen, C. A., Garetto, L. P., and Akeson, W. H.: The wick catheter technique for measurement of intramuscular pressure: a new research and clinical tool. J. Bone Joint Surg. 58-A:1016–1020, 1976.

Mubarak, S. J., and Owen, C. A.: Compartment syndrome and its relation to the crush syndrome: a spectrum of disease. Clin. Orthop. 113:81–89, 1975.

Mubarak, S. J., Owen, C. A., Hargens, A. R., Garetto, L. P., and Akeson, W. H.: Acute compartment syndromes: diagnosis and treatment with the aid of the wick catheter. J. Bone Joint Surg. 60-A:1091–1095, 1978B.

Murphy, J. B.: Myositis. J.A.M.A. 63:1249–1255, 1914.

Oberc, M. A., and Engel, W. K.: Ultrastructural localization of calcium in normal and abnormal skeletal muscle. Lab. Invest. 36:566–577, 1977.

Owen, C. A., Mubarak, S. J., Hargens, A. R., Rutherford, L., Garetto, L. P., and Akeson, W. H.: Intramuscular pressure with limb compression. Clarification of the pathogenesis of the drug-induced compartment syndrome/crush syndrome. N. Engl. J. Med. 300:1169–1172, 1979.

Patman, R. D., and Thompson, J. E.: Fasciotomy in peripheral vascular surgery. Arch. Surg. 101:663–672, 1970.

Reimer, K. A., Martonffy, K., Schumacher, B. L., Henkin, R. E., Quinn, J. L., III, and Jennings, R. B.: Localization of ^{99m}Tc-labeled pyrophosphate and calcium in myocardial infarcts after temporary coronary occlusion in dogs. Proc. Soc. Exp. Biol. Med. 156:272–276, 1977.

Reneman, R. S.: The Anterior and the Lateral Compartment Syndrome of The Leg. Mouton, The Hague, 1968, 176 pp.

Reneman, R. S., Slaaf, D. W., Lindbom, L., Tangelder, G. J., and Arfors, K-E.: Muscle blood flow disturbances produced by simultaneously elevated venous and total muscle tissue pressure. Microvasc. Res., 20:307–318, 1980.

Reneman, R. S., Slaaf, D. W., Lindbom, L., Tangelder, G. J., and Arfors, K-E.: Muscle blood flow disturbances in compartment syndromes and the role of elevated total muscle-tissue pressure in these disturbances. *In* Hargens, A. R. (ed.): Tissue Fluid Pressure and Composition. Williams and Wilkins Co., Baltimore, 1981, pp. 209–214.

Rorabeck, C. H., and Clarke, K. M.: The pathophysiology of the anterior tibial compartment syndrome: an experimental investigation. J. Trauma 18:299–304, 1978.

Rorabeck, C. H., and MacNab, I.: The pathophysiology of the anterior tibial compartmental syndrome. Clin. Orthop. 113:52–57, 1975.

Ryder, H. W., Molle, W. E.,and Ferris, E. B., Jr.: The influence of the collapsibility of veins on venous pressure, including a new procedure for measuring tissue pressure. J. Clin. Invest. 23:333–341, 1944.

Scully, R. E., Shannon, J. M., and Dickersin, G. R.: Factors involved in recovery from experimental skeletal muscle ischemia produced in dogs. I. Histologic and histochemical pattern of ischemic muscle. Am. J. Pathol. 39:721–734, 1961.

Shen, A. C., and Jennings, R. B.: Myocardial calcium and magnesium in acute ischemic injury. Am. J. Pathol. 67:417–440, 1972.

Sheridan, G. W., and Matsen, F. A., III: An animal model of the compartmental syndrome. Clin. Orthop. 113:36–42, 1975.

Sheridan, G. W., Matsen, F. A., III, and Krugmire, R. B., Jr.: Further investigations on the pathophysiology of the compartmental syndrome. Clin. Orthop. 123:266–270, 1977.

Shires, G. T., Cunningham, J. N., Baker, C. R. F., Reeder, S. F., Illner, H., Wagner, I. Y., and Maher, J.: Alterations in cellular membrane function during hemorrhagic shock in primates. Am. Surg. 176:288–295, 1972.

Smith, R. K., Tipton, C. M., Hargens, A. R., Evans, K. L., Zweifach, S. S., Gomez, M. A., Garfin, S. R., Mubarak, S. J., and Akeson, W. H.: Evaluation of long-term function in skeletal muscle. Orthop. Trans. 4:189, 1980.

Thomas, H. B.: Some orthopedic findings in ninety-eight cases of hemophilia. J. Bone Joint Surg. 18:140–147, 1936.

Vargas, F. F., and Johnson, J. A.: Effect of hyperosmolarity on resting and developed tension in heart muscle. Am. J. Physiol. 232:C155–C162, 1977.

Vogt, P. R.: Ischemic muscular necrosis following marching. Oregon State Med. Soc., Sept 4, 1943.

Volkmann, R. von: Die ischaemischen Muskellahmungen und Kontrakturen. Zentralb. Chir. 8:801–803, 1881.

Whitesides, T. E., Jr.: Compartment syndromes. Orthopedic Instruction Course, Am. Acad. Orthop. Surg., Dallas, Tx, 1978.

Whitesides, T. E., Jr., Haney, T. C., Morimoto, K., and Hirada, H.: Tissue pressure measurements as a determinant for the need of fasciotomy. Clin. Orthop. 113:43–51, 1975.

Whitesides, T. E., Jr., Harada, H., and Morimoto, K.: The response of skeletal muscle to temporary ischemia: an experimental study. Proc. Am. Acad. Orthop. Surg., J. Bone Joint Surg. 53-A:1027–1028, 1971.

Whitesides, T. E., Jr., Harada, H., and Morimoto, K.: Compartment syndromes and the role of fasciotomy, their parameters and techniques. Kappa Delta Award Paper No. 3, Am. Acad. Orthop. Surg., 47th Ann. Meeting, Atlanta, GA, Feb. 7, 1980.

Zweifach, S. S., Hargens, A. R., Evans, K. L., Gonsalves, M. R., Smith, R. K., Mubarak, S. J., and Akeson, W. H.: Skeletal muscle necrosis in pressurized compartments associated with hemorrhagic hypotension. J. Trauma 20:941–947, 1980.

Chapter Five

ETIOLOGIES OF COMPARTMENT SYNDROMES

Scott J. Mubarak, M.D.

A wide variety of injuries may initiate a compartment syndrome. Literature reviews on compartment syndrome and Volkmann's contracture in children and adults examine the most frequent causes of the problem (Table 5–1).

CHILDREN

The supracondylar fracture of the humerus in the child is the most infamous injury associated with a Volkmann's contracture. Increased awareness and therapeutic modifications of these fractures (D'Ambrosia, 1972; Dodge, 1972; Flynn et al., 1974) have reduced the frequency of this complication (Lipscomb, 1956; Eichler and Lipscomb, 1967; Mubarak and Carroll, 1979). Mubarak and Carroll (1979) reviewed the causes of Volkmann's contracture in 58 children and found that fractures predominated (Fig. 5–1). Thirty-six per cent of all Volkmann's contractures were caused by femur fracture, usually following inappropriate selection of traction technique. Supracondylar fractures still remained a frequent cause (16 per cent), although in our prospective study of acute compartment syndromes we have documented only one case in association with a supracondylar fracture and an arterial injury.

ADULTS

Bradley (1973) reviewed the world's literature and found that 38 per cent of all compartment syndromes dealt with arterial injuries and postischemic swelling, whereas 33 per cent were exercise-initiated syndromes (Table 5–1). Only 19 per cent were due to trauma. This review is misleading, as exercise-induced and postischemic problems tend to be reported much more frequently than fracture-induced compartment syndromes. A more accurate assessment was published by Sheridan and Matsen (1976), whose three most common causes of an acute

Table 5-1 MOST FREQUENT CAUSES REPORTED OF ACUTE COMPARTMENT SYNDROME OR VOLKMANN'S CONTRACTURE

Review CASES / Subject	Lipscomb (1956) 92 Volkmann's Contractures	Eichler and Lipscomb (1967) 32 Volkmann's Contractures	Bradley (1973) 137 Acute Compartment Syndromes	Sheridan and Matsen (1976) 44 Acute Compartment Syndromes	Mubarak and Carroll (1979) 58 Volkmann's Contractures	Mubarak and Hargens (1980)* 80 Acute Compartment Syndromes
1.	Supracondylar Fractures 48%	Supracondylar Fractures 34%	Postischemic Swelling 38%	Fractures 32%	Femur Fractures 36%	Fractures 45%
2.	Forearm Fractures 20%	Forearm Fractures 22%	Exercise 33%	Soft-Tissue Injury 14%	Supracondylar Fractures 16%	Soft-Tissue Injury 16%
3.	Humerus Fractures 8%	Soft-Tissue Injury 9%	Trauma 19%	Postischemic Swelling 14%	Forearm Fractures 16%	Postischemic Swelling 13%
4.	Postischemic Swelling 8%	Humerus Fractures 6%	Miscellaneous 26%	Gunshot 9%	Tibial Fractures 9%	Drug Overdose-Limb Compression 11%
5.	Elbow Dislocation 4%	Postischemic Swelling 3%	—	Intra-arterial Injection 9%	Postischemic Swelling 7%	Burns 5%
6.	Miscellaneous 12%	Miscellaneous 26%	—	Miscellaneous 22%	Miscellaneous 16%	Miscellaneous 10%
COMMENTS	Upper Extremity Only	Upper Extremity Only	Review of Literature	Retrospective Study	Children Only	Prospective Study

*Mubarak, S. J., and Hargens, A. R., unpublished data, 1980.

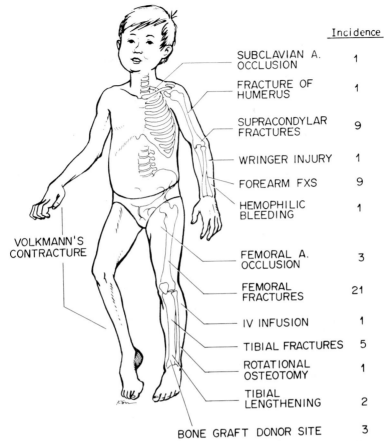

	Incidence
SUBCLAVIAN A. OCCLUSION	1
FRACTURE OF HUMERUS	1
SUPRACONDYLAR FRACTURES	9
WRINGER INJURY	1
FOREARM FXS	9
HEMOPHILIC BLEEDING	1
FEMORAL A. OCCLUSION	3
FEMORAL FRACTURES	21
IV INFUSION	1
TIBIAL FRACTURES	5
ROTATIONAL OSTEOTOMY	1
TIBIAL LENGTHENING	2
BONE GRAFT DONOR SITE	3

VOLKMANN'S CONTRACTURE

Figure 5–1 Causes of Volkmann's contracture in 58 limbs (55 children). (With permission from Mubarak, S. J., and Carroll, N. C.: Volkmann's contracture in children: aetiology and prevention. J Bone Joint Surg 61-B:285–293, 1979.)

compartment syndrome (fractures, soft-tissue injury, and postischemic swelling) are identical to the primary causes in our experience.

We have studied over 80 cases prospectively using the wick catheter. By far the most common cause of an acute compartment syndrome is fracture (45 per cent), the majority being fractures of the tibia (Fig. 5–2). Soft-tissue injury accounted for 16 per cent, and arterial injury with postischemic swelling for 13 per cent in this series. The drug overdose-limb compression group of patients constituted 11 per cent. Surprisingly, 85 per cent of these cases have occurred in the lower extremity.

We have modified Matsen's classification (1975) and will discuss the various etiologies. These can be subdivided into problems that (1) decrease the size of the compartment or (2) increase the fluid content in the compartment. In the second group, the fluid that accumulates may be primarily edema, hemorrhage, or a combination of edema and hemorrhage (Table 5–2).

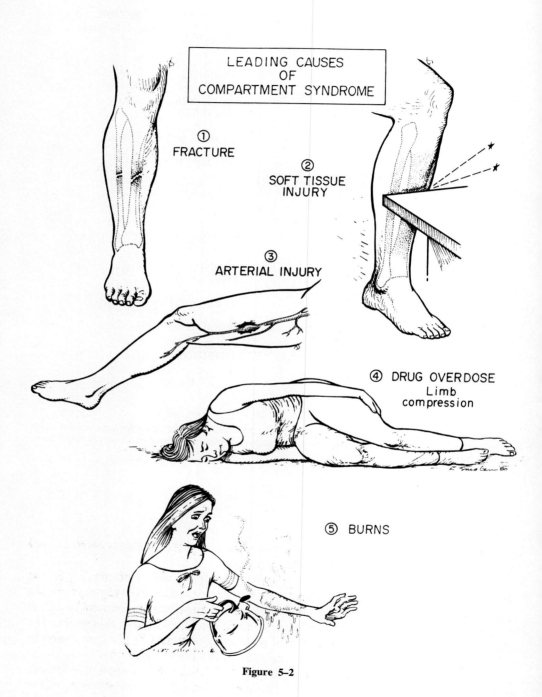

LEADING CAUSES
OF
COMPARTMENT SYNDROME

① FRACTURE

② SOFT TISSUE INJURY

③ ARTERIAL INJURY

④ DRUG OVERDOSE
Limb compression

⑤ BURNS

Figure 5–2

Table 5–2 CLASSIFICATION OF ACUTE COMPARTMENT SYNDROMES

Decreased Compartment Size
1. Constrictive Dressings and Casts
2. Closure of Fascial Defects
3. Thermal Injuries and Frostbite

Increased Compartment Contents

PRIMARILY EDEMA ACCUMULATION
1. Postischemic Swelling
   a. Arterial Injuries
   b. Arterial Thrombosis or Embolism
   c. Reconstructive Vascular and Bypass Surgery
   d. Replantation
   e. Prolonged Tourniquet Time
   f. Arterial Spasm
   g. Cardiac Catheterization and Angiography
   h. Ergotamine Ingestion
2. Prolonged Immobilization with Limb Compression
   a. Drug Overdose with Limb Compression
   b. General Anesthesia with Knee-Chest Position
3. Thermal Injuries and Frostbite
4. Exertion
5. Venous Disease
6. Venomous Snakebite

PRIMARILY HEMORRHAGE ACCUMULATION
1. Hereditary Bleeding Disorders, e.g., Hemophilia
2. Anticoagulant Therapy
3. Vessel Laceration

COMBINATION OF EDEMA AND HEMORRHAGE ACCUMULATION
1. Fractures
   a. Tibia
   b. Forearm
   c. Elbow, e.g., Supracondylar
   d. Femur
2. Soft-Tissue Injury
3. Osteotomies, e.g., Tibia

MISCELLANEOUS
1. Intravenous Infiltration, e.g., Blood, Saline
2. Popliteal Cyst
3. Long Leg Brace

DECREASED COMPARTMENT SIZE

CONSTRICTIVE DRESSINGS AND CASTS

The effects of casts and circular dressings on restriction of compartment size and swelling are discussed in detail in Chapter 8. Obviously, an injury that requires a cast is an integral part of the compartment syndrome pathogenesis. The cast lowers tissue compliance, and thus also lowers the threshold of fluid accumulation that will elevate the pressure to ischemic levels in the compartment.

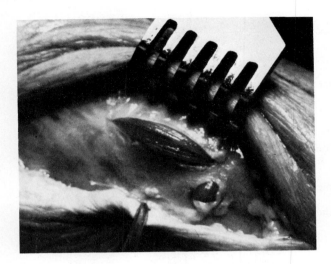

Figure 5–3 Closure of fascial defects may precipitate an acute compartment syndrome.

CLOSURE OF FASCIAL DEFECTS

Sirbu and associates (1944) were the first to report on closure of a fascial defect in the leg and the ensuing ischemic complication. Since then, other case reports documenting this problem have been published (Leach et al., 1967, Paton, 1968; Wolfort et al., 1973). The appearance of a muscle hernia and fascial defect is the result of increased pressure in the underlying compartment (Fig. 5–3). These muscle hernias are seen most often in patients with symptoms of a chronic exertional compartment syndrome (see Chapter 14). Closure of this defect causes a decrease in the volume of the compartment and, as has been reported, an acute compartment syndrome can then occur. Reports in the literature indicate that this acute compartment syndrome presents within hours to days following the closure of the fascial defect (Sirbu et al., 1944; Paton, 1968; Wolfort et al., 1973). Accordingly, closure of fascial defects in the leg or forearm is never indicated.

THERMAL INJURIES AND FROSTBITE

A circumferential, third-degree burn causes a type of acute compartment syndrome for two reasons. First, the inelastic, constricting eschar decreases the volume of the underlying compartments; second, thermal injuries are associated with an obligatory edema formation. Many authors have reported on the value of escharotomy (decompression of the underlying tissues by division of the burned skin, subcutaneous and fascial layers) in the treatment of burns (Moncrief, 1969; Patman and Thompson, 1970). Pruitt and associates (1968) reviewed 485 burn cases, in 11 per cent of which escharotomy was performed. Justis et al. (1976) reported four cases of acute compartment syndromes of the leg that resulted from burns. In only one case was early surgical decompression employed. Similarly, in high-voltage electrical burns of the limbs, early surgical decompression is indicated (Mann and Wallquist, 1975). These authors noted that in eight cases there was decreased patient morbidity and earlier rehabilitation after escharotomy. In a pathologic study of 29 consecutive autopsies of burn patients (Salisbury et al., 1974), 62 per cent showed evidence of necrosis in the intrinsic muscles of the hand resulting from untreated compartment syndromes.

With burn injuries the usual parameters of sensory loss, pain with stretch, and even the palpation of compartment tightness are lost owing to the severity of the thermal injury. Evaluation of the peripheral pulses, even with Doppler techniques, as an indication for decompression would mean waiting for a critical pressure level that is too high (arterial systolic pressure). In a prospective study, Suffee and collaborators (1979) used wick catheters to measure intracompartmental pressures in burn victims. They correlated the underlying pressure with the percentage of body surface area injured. Nine of 16 patients with more than 30 per cent burns had pressures in the extremities greater than 30 mm Hg. Furthermore, the elevated pressures (greater than 30 mm Hg) were seen only after circumferential burns of the limbs. We concur with these findings, and suggest further that the use of tissue pressure measurement is invaluable in third-degree burns to evaluate the need for decompression.

Pathologic changes and edema formation similar to those in thermal injuries, occur after frostbite. Fasciotomy has been advocated in frostbite injuries (Fowler and Willis, 1975; Franz et al., 1978).

INCREASED COMPARTMENT CONTENTS

Edema Accumulation

POSTISCHEMIC SWELLING

Compartment syndromes or Volkmann's contracture are commonly associated with arterial injuries or thrombosis. Griffiths (1940) was one of the first to relate arterial injuries to Volkmann's contracture, although he confused and combined the findings of a compartment syndrome with those of an arterial injury. Starting with Sirbu and co-workers (1944), numerous examples of arterial injury, thrombosis, and embolism with subsequent compartment syndrome or Volkmann's contracture have been reported (Hughes, 1948; Horn and Sevitt, 1951; Watson, 1955; Harrison and Jackson, 1956; Kunkel and Lynn, 1958; Freedman and Knowles, 1959; Lytton and Blandy, 1960; Mozes et al., 1962; Tilney and McLamb, 1967; Coupland, 1972). The swelling that follows cardiac bypass, femoropopliteal bypass (Gitlitz, 1965), and replantation surgery (Eiken et al., 1964; Patman, 1975) also may initiate compartment syndromes. Most of these problems have occurred in the lower extremities. Of these causes, arterial injuries are much more likely to produce a compartment syndrome than is either venous injury, arterial embolization, or arterial reconstruction (Patman and Thompson, 1970) (Table 5–3). Rarely, mainline intra-arterial drug injection may precipitate a compartment syndrome (Morgan et al., 1970; Hawkins et al., 1973; Eaton and Green, 1975).

The necessity for fasciotomy after arterial injuries has been stressed by numerous authors since World War II (DeBakey and Simeone, 1946; Rich et al., 1969; Patman and Thompson, 1970; Jacob, 1974; Fowler and Willis, 1975; Kelly and Eiseman, 1975). The frequency of use of fasciotomy as a complementary procedure to arterial repair has varied from 6 and 7 per cent (Kelly and Eiseman, 1975; Jacob, 1974) to 33 per cent (Patman and Thompson, 1970).

An injury to a major artery may produce a compartment syndrome by two basic mechanisms. First, if complete arterial occlusion (arterial injury, thrombosis, or

Table 5–3 FREQUENCY OF USE OF FASCIOTOMY TO RELIEVE
COMPARTMENT SYNDROMES IN PERIPHERAL VASCULAR SURGERY*

Type of Injury	Total Number of Patients	Number of Patients Undergoing Fasciotomy	Percentage
Arterial Injuries	352	113	32
Venous Injury	51	7	14
Arterial Embolization	200	4	2
Arterial Reconstruction	2000	8	0.45
Replantation	1	1	100

*From Patman, R. D.: Compartmental syndromes in peripheral vascular surgery. Clin. Orthop. 113:103–110, 1975.

embolization) has been present long enough to produce ischemic changes, restoration of circulation to the damaged capillary bed and muscle may produce enough edema (postischemic swelling) to initiate a compartment syndrome. With complete arterial occlusion in which the circulation is not restored, gangrene, rather than a compartment syndrome, will result (Fig. 5–4). The total time of arterial ischemia is important. Whitesides and associates (1977) demonstrated that six hours of tourniquet-induced ischemia in dogs produced markedly elevated intracompartmental pressures after removal of the tourniquet. In similar canine tourniquet experiments, we have noted postischemic pressure greater than 50 mm Hg in some cases, with only four hours of tourniquet ischemia. Unless fasciotomy is performed at the time of arterial repair, the resulting postischemic compartment syndrome will prolong the period of ischemia to muscles and nerves of the compartment (Fig. 5–5). We therefore recommend routine fasciotomy after arterial repair if the ischemic period has been longer than six hours.

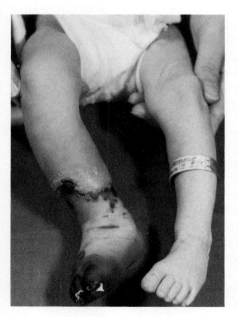

Figure 5–4 Newborn infant with right popliteal artery occlusion and distal gangrene. With complete arterial occlusion in which the circulation is not restored, gangrene rather than a compartment syndrome will result.

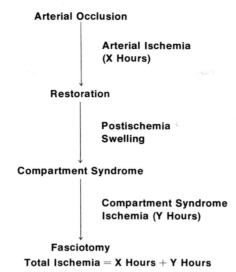

Arterial Occlusion

**Arterial Ischemia
(X Hours)**

Restoration

**Postischemia
Swelling**

Compartment Syndrome

**Compartment Syndrome
Ischemia (Y Hours)**

Fasciotomy
Total Ischemia = X Hours + Y Hours

Figure 5–5   Pathogenesis of postischemia-initiated compartment syndromes.

A less common mechanism of compartment syndrome pathogenesis may result if the artery is only partially occluded (e.g., an intimal tear) and there is inadequate collateral circulation. In this situation the decreased perfusion and ischemia of muscle capillaries will cause an increase in the permeability of the capillary walls. The resulting edema will cause more ischemia, and the self-perpetuating formation of a compartment syndrome will be established before arterial repair. Thus, in this circumstance, both the arterial injury and the compartment syndrome are present at the same time, and both will require immediate treatment.

In the years following World War I a number of authors brought attention to arterial spasm and subsequent gangrene (Küttner and Baruch, 1920; Montgomery and Ireland, 1935). Leriche (1928) was one of the first to associate Volkmann's ischemic contracture with arterial spasm. Griffiths (1940) then popularized the arterial injury and spasm concept, dismissing the works of Brookes (1922) and Jepson (1926) on venous occlusion and elevated intracompartmental pressure.

Arterial spasm can be induced experimentally by prolonged tourniquet use (Barnes and Trueta, 1942), increased intracompartmental pressure (Benjamin, 1957; Eaton and Green, 1972), and by soft-tissue injury and excessive traction (Mustard and Simmons, 1953). We have observed arterial spasm with elevated pressure in our canine compartment syndrome model, and clinically in exploring limbs or decompressing compartments, particularly in the young. Arterial spasm may play a role in the compartment syndrome cases that have resulted after cardiac catheterization (Rosengart et al., 1976), although embolization is probably the main factor following this procedure (Mubarak and Carroll, 1979).

Tissue pressure measurement and arteriograms have allowed physicians to evaluate the ischemic limbs more completely. In these cases arterial spasm is rarely, if ever, the primary diagnosis. Moreover, the necessity for treating arterial spasm remains enigmatic.

Drug-induced vasospasm has been reported as a cause of bilateral anterior compartment syndromes by Elliott and Glass (1976). In their case, excessive ingestion of ergotamine in the treatment of a migraine headache induced a peripheral arterial spasm of the patient's legs. After treatment of the ergotamine overdose, the postischemic swelling caused the compartment syndromes.

PROLONGED IMMOBILIZATION WITH LIMB COMPRESSION

Prolonged immobilization in patients after drug overdose or after a general anesthetic in the knee-chest position is a common cause of compartment syndromes and crush syndromes. The details of this condition are covered extensively in Chapter 11.

THERMAL INJURIES AND FROSTBITE

See the section on Decreased Compartment Size earlier in this chapter.

EXERTION

The exercise-initiated compartment syndromes are divided into two forms, acute and chronic, and are covered extensively in Chapter 14.

Excessive muscular contraction and spasm following seizures and androgen ingestion have been documented as etiologic factors. Halpern and Nagel (1977) reported a 32 year old woman with rheumatoid arthritis who developed problems following gold therapy that necessitated administration of prednisone and ox-ymetholone (an androgen compound). Forty-eight hours after this therapy had been initated the patient developed anterior and lateral compartment syndromes bilateral-ly that required decompression. These authors hypothesized that the androgen compound caused a spasm in the muscles and that this initiated the syndrome. Manson (1964) reported a patient who developed a compartment syndrome after a seizure lasting an hour and a half that was due to postpartum eclampsia. This patient also received ergotamine, which probably was an additive factor. Lees (1976) documented a case arising from prolonged tetany following hypocalcemia and respiratory alkalosis. Caldwell (1957) and Fowler and Willis (1975) noted cases following seizures. All these cases have prolonged seizuring and excessive muscle exertion in common.

VENOUS DISEASE

In the 1920s both Brookes (1922) and Jepson (1926) used venous occlusion experimentally in animals to produce massive limb swelling and the pathologic changes of Volkmann's contracture. However, in clinical cases, venous injury or thrombosis remains an uncommon cause of a compartment syndrome except in its more severe form, phlegmasia cerulea dolens (venous gangrene).

Phlegmasia cerulea dolens is a relatively rare condition of venous thrombosis with massive distal swelling. Seventy-five per cent of cases are in the lower

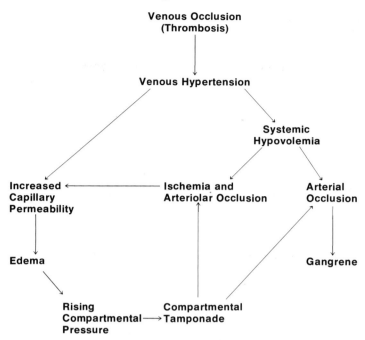

Figure 5–6 Presumed pathogenesis of compartment syndrome and arterial occlusion resulting from phlegmasia cerulea dolens (venous occlusion).

extremities. Arterial insufficiency and gangrene are frequently associated with this disorder. The former is probably a result of a systemic hypovolemia and the high intracompartmental pressure. The presumed mechanism of compartment syndrome pathogenesis and arterial occlusion is illustrated in Figure 5–6.

Severe pain, more intense than with thrombophlebitis, is present with phlegmasia cerulea dolens. Other findings are dusky skin and petechial hemorrhages, along with massive swelling. Pulses, present initially, are usually lost.

The treatment is variable and in dispute. Sympathetic blocks, elevation, exercise, anticoagulants, and thrombectomy have all been used. Decompression was first demonstrated by Dennis (1945) to be of value in this disorder. He employed decompression based on experimental results of fasciotomies that Jepson described in 1926. Since then, Cywes and Louw (1962) and Patman and Thompson (1970) have been strong advocates for early fasciotomy along with thrombectomy and postural drainage for cases of phlegmasia cerulea dolens.

VENOMOUS SNAKEBITE

The existence of compartment syndromes and the need for fasciotomy following pit viper envenomation are in much dispute. In over 550 cases treated or followed, Russell et al. (1975) have not seen one case that required decompression or that resulted in a Volkmann's contracture after appropriate medical treatment. Refuting this evidence, Glass (1976) and others (Henderson and Dujon, 1973; Huang et al., 1974; Patman, 1975; Grace et al., 1978) believe that a presumed intramuscular injection of venom requires immediate fasciotomy in most, if not all, pit viper bites. From analysis of the literature, however, it is difficult to conclude whether compartment syndromes do or do not occur following rattlesnake bites. Except for our studies (Garfin et al., 1979B), no cases have been documented with pressure studies, and most descriptions of compartment contents after fasciotomy are vague.

Even with subcutaneous envenomation, the clinical findings mimic those of an acute compartment syndrome. The involved extremities are dusky, ecchymotic, edematous, and extremely tender. Dysesthesias as well as spotty areas of anesthesia are present. Motor function is diminished, and passive stretch of the involved muscle causes severe pain. These signs are identical to those seen in acute compartment syndromes, but can also be explained by the venom's neurotoxic and tissue-destroying enzymes.

Experimentally, we have studied the effects of snake venom on canine hind limbs. Desiccated crotalid venom (3 mg) was injected at various depths into canine hind limbs through a syringe and 23-gauge needle. Subcutaneous injections superficial to the anterolateral compartment were done in six limbs. In ten limbs the venom was deposited within the anterolateral compartment, and in six limbs it was injected into the muscles of the compartment after fasciectomy had been performed and the skin closed. Subcutaneous and intracompartmental pressures were recorded with wick catheters in all limbs. After 48 hours the dogs were sacrificed, and subcutaneous and intracompartmental tissues were examined macroscopically and microscopically (Garfin et al., 1979A).

The limbs of each envenomated dog appeared grossly identical in terms of edema and ecchymoses. Hind-limb circumferences and temperature rose equally, regardless of the depth of injection. Increases in intracompartmental pressure were observed only after direct muscular envenomations. Pressures rose significantly about two hours after envenomation, with an average maximal intracompartmental pressure of 84 ± 10 mm Hg at 20 hours (Table 5–4). When a fasciectomy was performed prior to envenomation, the pressure did not exceed 30 mm Hg.

Histologically, the muscles in all limbs envenomated intracompartmentally were uniformly necrotic, with large areas of hemorrhage and acute inflammation. No

Table 5–4   RESULTS: INJECTION OF RATTLESNAKE VENOM INTO CANINE HIND LIMBS (NUMBER = 22)*

INJECTION	Pressures (mm Hg) SUBCUTANEOUS	INTRA-COMPARTMENTAL	△ SURFACE TEMPERATURE (C)	△ LEG CIRCUMFERENCE (CM)
Subcutaneous	5 ± 1	7 ± 1	2.4 ± 1.2	3.25 ± 1.63
Intramuscular	4 ± 2	84 ± 10**	1.6 ± 0.59	3.57 ± 0.45
Postfasciectomy intramuscular		20 ± 2**		

Values are mean ± SE.
*Modified from Garfin, S. R., et al.: Role of surgical decompression in treatment of rattlesnake bites. Surg., Forum. 30:502–504, 1979A.
**The difference in intracompartmental pressure with and without fasciectomy is statistically significant (P < 0.005).

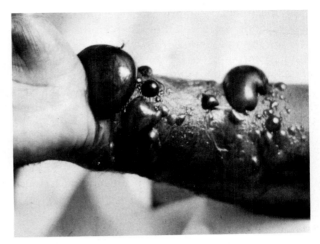

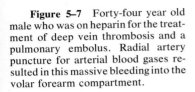

Figure 5–7 Forty-four year old male who was on heparin for the treatment of deep vein thrombosis and a pulmonary embolus. Radial artery puncture for arterial blood gases resulted in this massive bleeding into the volar forearm compartment.

difference was observed between compartments with or without fasciectomy. When the venom was deposited subcutaneously the contents of the compartment appeared normal, except for peripheral areas of leukocyte infiltration and inflammation. These latter dogs had no elevation of compartmental pressure (Garfin et al., 1979A).

Our conclusions from this study are twofold. First, if the bite is subcutaneous, muscular involvement is minimal and surgical decompression appears to be unwarranted. Second, although fasciectomy decreased intracompartmental pressure, muscle destruction by the venom was not prevented.

Clinically, we have found that only one of a dozen patients we have studied had intracompartmental pressures above the critical level necessitating fasciotomy (>30 mm Hg). This experience has led us to adopt a primarily medical mode of management for rattlesnake venom poisoning, and to de-emphasize routine surgical decompression.

Hemorrhage Accumulation

Hey Groves (1907) was the first to describe a Volkmann's contracture in association with hemophilia. Hill and Brookes (1936) and Thomas (1936) reviewed more cases on this subject, and discussed their pathogenesis. Lancourt et al. (1977) reported 34 complications of hemophilia in the hand and forearm, four of which involved a Volkmann's contracture. These authors recommended fasciotomy, but did not employ it in the treatment of their patients.

Acute compartment syndromes have been reported as complications of arterial punctures in anticoagulated patients (Luce et al., 1976; Neviaser et al., 1976; Halpern et al., 1978). In all these cases the patients were on therapeutic doses of either heparin or warfarin products, and following arterial puncture to determine blood gases in the radial, brachial, or femoral artery, massive bleeding occurred with a resulting compartment syndrome (Fig. 5–7).

The iliacus syndrome with a femoral neuropathy has been described in association with both hemophilia (Brower and Wilde, 1966; Goodfellow et al., 1967) and anticoagulant therapy (Wells and Templeton, 1977). Bleeding in the iliacus "compartment" compromises the function of the femoral nerve. This syndrome is discussed in more detail in Chapter 10.

Even in patients with normal clotting studies, bleeding may initiate a compartment syndrome. We have noted two cases of a syndrome developing as an isolated injury from a stab wound to a major artery of the forearm.

In our experience during decompression of hemorrhage-initiated compartment syndromes, whether it be from vessel laceration or a bleeding diasthesis, we have noted a moderate amount of edema in the muscles, and therefore do not advise immediate closure after evacuation of the hematoma.

Combination of Edema and Hemorrhage Accumulation

FRACTURES

Fractures represent the most common cause of an acute compartment syndrome, in our experience: specifically, fractures of the tibia. The incidence of Volkmann's contracture following tibial shaft fractures ranges from 3 per cent (Ellis, 1958) to 10 per cent (Owen and Tsimboukis, 1967). Rorabeck and MacNab (1976)

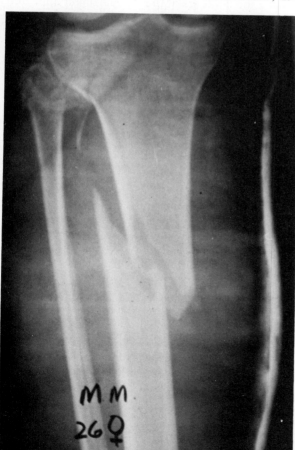

Figure 5–8 Closed as well as open tibial fractures are the most common cause of an acute compartment syndrome.

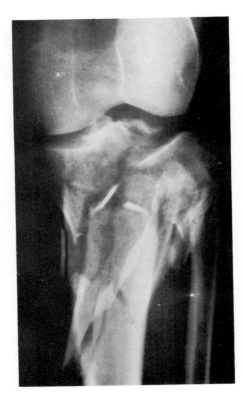

Figure 5–9 Tibial plateau fractures are frequently associated with either an acute compartment syndrome or a peroneal nerve injury.

have reported the largest series of syndromes caused by tibial fractures (25 cases). We have noted acute compartment syndrome after fractures of the tibial plateau, diaphysis, and ankle. Furthermore, open as well as closed tibial fractures can be associated with an acute compartment syndrome (Figs. 5–8 to 5–10).

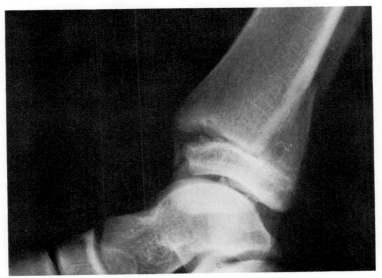

Figure 5–10 This adolescent boy developed anterior and lateral compartment syndromes following this epiphyseal separation of the distal tibia.

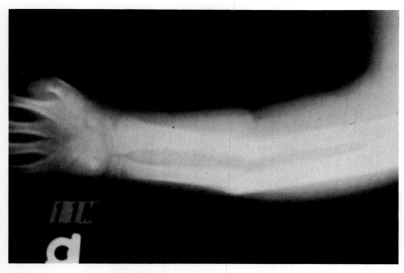

Figure 5–11 This 11 year old boy sustained volar and dorsal compartment syndromes following a fracture of both bones of the forearm.

Forearm fractures in both adults (Gelberman et al., 1980) and children (Mubarak and Carroll, 1979) represent a common cause of forearm compartment syndromes. These vary from radial head fractures or epiphyseal separations of the distal radius (Mubarak and Carroll, 1979) to segmental fractures of the radius and ulna (Figs. 5–11, 5–12).

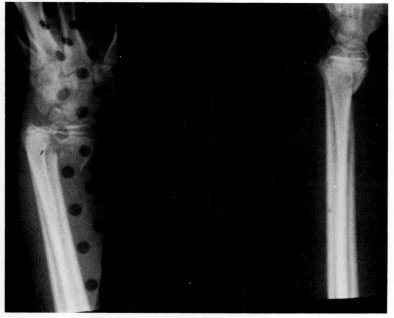

Figure 5–12 Epiphyseal separations of the distal radius may also result in an acute compartment syndrome.

Fractures of the humerus or femur in association with acute compartment syndromes or Volkmann's contracture are type I injuries, according to the classification of Holden (1975). In this classification, type I injuries occur above the knee or elbow, with subsequent ischemia developing distal to the knee or elbow. Most type I injuries are associated with injuries to a major artery. In type II the direct trauma to the limb and subsequent ischemia occur at the same site (below the elbow or below the knee). Fractures of the tibia or forearm are examples of type II injuries.

The classic example of a type I injury is the supracondylar fracture of the distal humerus in the child (Figs. 5–13, 5–14). Injury to the brachial artery is common, and ranges from 8 to 18 per cent (D'Ambrosia, 1972; Dodge, 1972; Flynn et al., 1974) with this fracture. The compartment syndrome develops from postischemic swelling or from the hemorrhage and edema of the initial injury. Fortunately, as mentioned previously, compartment syndromes and Volkmann's contracture are rarely seen today with the treatment modalities currently used for supracondylar fractures.

The ischemia that follows a femoral fracture in a child (type I injury) may be due to a compartment syndrome, an arterial injury, inappropriate use of traction, or a combination of these. Femoral fractures also are occasionally associated with arterial injuries (Grosz et al., 1973). The arterial injury must be recognized early, and when circulation is restored, fasciotomy must be considered (Fig. 5–15).

Compartment syndromes associated with femoral fractures treated with Bryant's traction in children were reported by Winslow (1950) and Thomson and Mahoney (1951) (Fig. 5–16). Nicholson et al. (1955) believed that the primary factors that caused impaired circulation in children treated with Bryant's traction were the

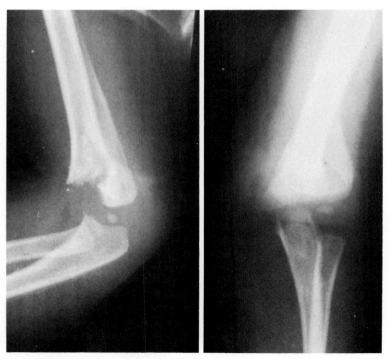

Figure 5–13 The supracondylar fracture of the distal humerus in a child is the most infamous fracture associated with Volkmann's contracture. This three year old boy's supracondylar fracture was well healed at six weeks postinjury.

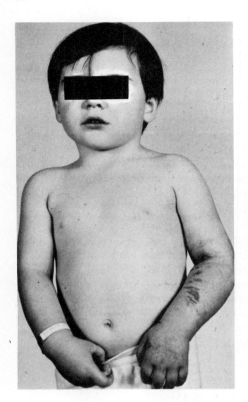

Figure 5–14 Three year old boy whose supracondylar fracture is shown in Figure 5–13. At the time of cast removal his forearm was noted to have poor sensation and to be contracted in the pronated and flexed position. All supracondylar fractures must be evaluated carefully for arterial injury, nerve injury, and compartment syndromes.

Figure 5–15 This closed femoral fracture in a four year old girl was associated with an arterial injury. Delay in recognition of the arterial injury and no treatment of the postischemic compartment syndrome resulted in significant functional loss in the leg.

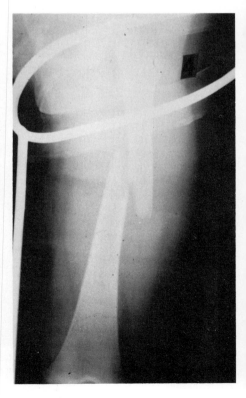

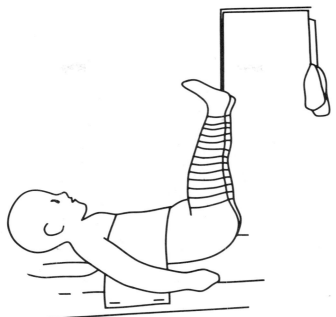

Figure 5–16 Volkmann's contracture resulting from femoral fractures treated with Bryant's traction in children can occur even in the uninjured limb. This traction should not be used for any child over two years of age or over 30 pounds in weight.

reduction in hydrostatic pressure in the lower limbs held in the overhead position, aggravated by tight bandaging, shock, traction, and hyperextension of the knee. When placing a child in Bryant's traction, care should be taken in wrapping the leg and in avoiding hyperextension of the knee. Frequent neurovascular checks of the feet are mandatory. Bryant's traction should not be used for any child over two years of age or over 30 pounds in weight (Mubarak and Carroll, 1979).

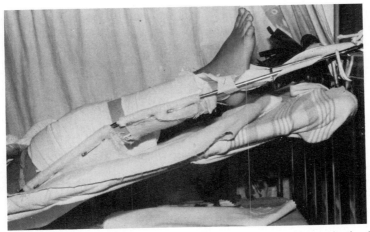

Figure 5–17 Femoral fractures in the older child may be treated with skin traction in a Thomas splint elevated on a Bradford frame, but careful and frequent neurovascular examinations must be performed.

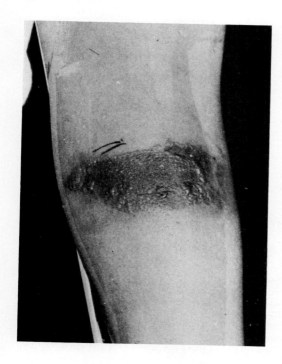

Figure 5–18 This patient developed an acute, superficial, posterior compartment syndrome following a closed femoral fracture. He was treated with skin traction in a Thomas splint on a Bradford frame. Note the erythema and pressure blisters overlying the calf musculature.

Thomson and Mahoney (1951) first associated Volkmann's contracture and femoral fractures in an older child who was immobilized with skin traction in a Thomas splint and elevated on a Bradford frame (Fig. 5–17). They documented eight cases of Volkmann's contracture, to which Mubarak and Carroll (1979) added an additional 11 examples. The presenting complex of symptoms consists of severe pain in the calf, aggravated by dorsiflexion of the ankle that occurs 12 to 48 hours postinjury. The skin over a tense calf is erythematous, and "pressure blisters" are occasionally present (Fig. 5–18). Rarely, diminished pulses and decreased sensation in the distribution of the sural nerve are also noted. The mechanism of injury is probably a combination of arterial spasm or injury, elevation of the leg, and direct pressure over the superficial posterior compartment from the traction apparatus. Careful and frequent neurovascular examination of children treated with this form of traction is mandatory.

SOFT-TISSUE INJURY

In our experience, the second leading cause of a compartment syndrome is severe soft-tissue injury or contusion without an associated fracture. In many cases this may represent a crushing trauma, but we have noted acute compartment syndromes following a rather minor blunt trauma over the anterior compartment of the leg or the volar compartment of the forearm (Figs. 5–19 to 5–21).

Crushing injuries to limbs, whether produced by debris or machinery, are a primary cause of compartment and crush syndromes (Fig. 5–22). Bywaters and Beall (1941) first brought attention to this symptom complex during World War II.

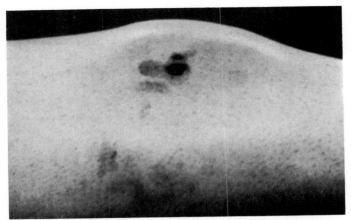

Figure 5–19 Patient E. I., a 24 year old male who sustained a contusion and this tiny puncture wound to the anterior compartment of the left leg. The clinical examination on admission demonstrated decreased sensation in the superficial and deep peroneal nerve distribution.

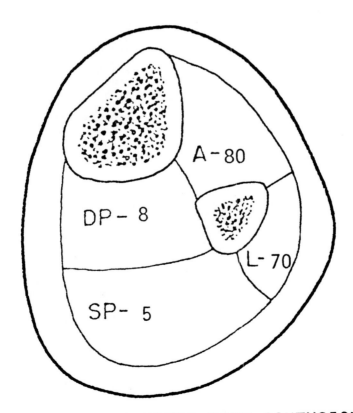

E.I. - 4 HOURS POST CONTUSION

Figure 5–20 Patient E. I. had wick catheter pressure studies performed four hours postinjury to differentiate between peroneal nerve contusion and acute compartment syndrome. The anterior and lateral compartment pressures were markedly elevated.

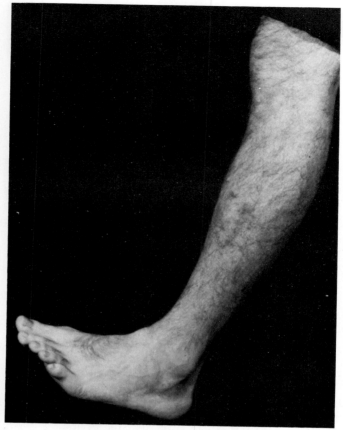

Figure 5–21   Patient E. I. six months postfasciotomy of the anterior and lateral compartments. The wound is well healed, he has normal sensation, and, as demonstrated, dorsiflexion power of the foot and ankle is normal.

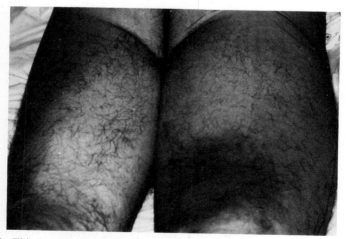

Figure 5–22   This 25 year old male sustained a crushing injury to the right posterior thigh. Initial evaluation revealed no fractures, normal sensation, marked pain, and a rather tense hamstrings compartment. Maximal intracompartmental pressure measurement was 25 mm Hg. The patient was kept under observation and gradually the swelling resolved. One month following this injury there was normal function without neurologic residual.

Occasionally one sees cases of machinery or debris crushing a limb and initiating this problem today (see Chapter 11).

Wringer injuries from washing machines are much less frequent nowadays and are not a common cause of a compartment syndrome (Stone et al., 1976; Mubarak and Carroll, 1979).

OSTEOTOMIES OF THE TIBIA

Osteotomies of the tibia in children and adults sometimes produce acute compartment syndromes (Schrock, 1969; Steel et al., 1971; Jackson and Waugh, 1974; Matsen and Staheli, 1975) (Fig. 5–23). Transfer of the tibial tubercle for recurrent dislocation of the patella (Hauser procedure) has also been associated with acute compartment syndromes and Volkmann's contracture (Wiggins, 1975; Wall, 1979). Mubarak and Carroll (1979) noted three cases of Volkmann's contracture of the leg in children in whom the tibia was used as a source for bone graft. Furthermore, in that same review, two cases of tibial lengthening were associated with acute compartment syndromes. The literature fairly accurately documents the high association of operations on the tibia with acute compartment syndromes (Fig. 5–24).

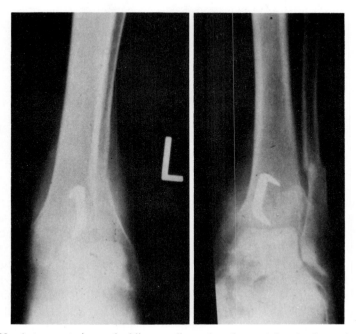

Figure 5–23 Anteroposterior and oblique radiographs of an adolescent boy who underwent a derotation osteotomy of the distal tibia for a residual clubfoot deformity. He subsequently developed acute compartment syndromes of this leg, and the resulting Volkmann's contracture and its neurologic residual necessitated Syme amputation.

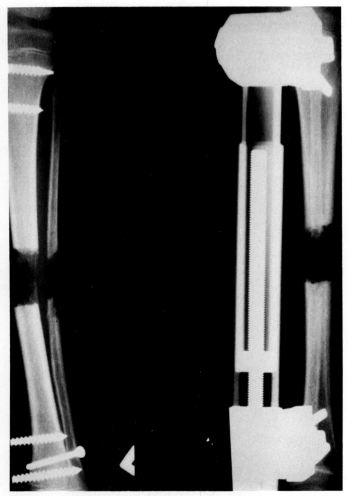

Figure 5–24 Tibia leg-lengthening procedures may be associated with acute compartment syndromes. After tibial osteotomy the anterior and lateral compartment fascia should be incised.

Miscellaneous

Intravenous infiltration of blood (Bowden and Gutman, 1949; Carter et al., 1949; Maor et al., 1972; Eaton and Green, 1975) and saline (Lipscomb, 1956; Mubarak and Carroll, 1979) into a compartment may cause a compartment syndrome.

Sweeney and O'Brien (1965) described a patient with the nephrotic syndrome who developed bilateral anterior compartment syndromes. They theorized that peripheral edema secondary to the nephrotic syndrome, recent leg trauma, and atherosclerotic vascular disease were additional factors in initiating this problem.

Other unusual cases reported in the literature involved internal or external pressure. A deep posterior compartment syndrome may result from a dissecting popliteal cyst (Scott et al., 1977). Even more unusual, a 20 month old boy using a brace for genu varum developed an anterior compartment syndrome (Weitz and Carson, 1969). These latter authors hypothesized that there was excessive pressure from the brace over the anterior compartment.

In view of the wide variety of causes reported, nearly all subspecialties of medicine and surgery should be aware of the compartment syndrome. In particular, however, the specialties of orthopedics, vascular surgery, general surgery, and traumatology must be able to diagnosis and treat this entity expeditiously.

REFERENCES

Barnes, J. M., and Trueta, J.: Arterial spasm: an experimental study. Br. J. Surg 30:74–79, 1942.

Benjamin, A.: The relief of traumatic arterial spasm in threatened Volkmann's ischaemic contracture. J. Bone Joint Surg. 39-B:711–713, 1957.

Bowden, R. F. M., and Gutman, E.: The fate of voluntary muscle after vascular injury in man. J. Bone Joint Surg. 31-B:356–368, 1949.

Bradley, E. L.: The anterior tibial compartment syndrome. Surg. Gynecol. Obstet. 136:289–297, 1973.

Brookes, B.: Pathologic changes in muscle as a result of disturbances of circulation: an experimental study of Volkmann's ischemic paralysis. Arch. Surg. 5:188–216, 1922.

Brower, T. D., and Wilde, A. H.: Femoral neuropathy in hemophilia. J. Bone Joint Surg. 48-A:487–492, 1966.

Bywaters, E. G. L., and Beall, D.: Crush injuries with impairment of renal function. Br. Med. J. 1:427–434, 1941.

Caldwell, R. K.: Ischemic necrosis of the anterior tibial muscle: case report with autopsy findings, and review of the literature. Ann. Intern. Med. 46:1191–1199, 1957.

Carter, A. B., Richard, R. L., and Zachary, R. B.: The anterior tibial syndrome. Lancet 2:928–934, 1949.

Coupland, G. A. E.: Anterior tibial syndrome following restoration of arterial flow. Aust. N. Z. J. Surg. 41:338–341, 1972.

Cywes, S., and Louw, J. G.: Phlegmasia cerulea dolens: successful treatment by relieving fasciotomy. Surgery 51:169–176, 1962.

D'Ambrosia, R. D.: Supracondylar fractures of the humerus: prevention of cubitus varus. J. Bone Joint Surg. 54-A:60–66, 1972.

DeBakey, M. E., and Simeone, F. A.: Battle injuries of the arteries in World War II. An analysis of 2,471 cases. Ann. Surg. 123:534–579, 1946.

Dennis, C.: Diaster following femoral vein ligation for thrombophlebitis; relief by fasciotomy; clinical case of renal impairment following crush injury. Surgery 17:264–269, 1945.

Dodge, H. S.: Displaced supracondylar fractures of the humerus in children: treatment by Dunlop's traction. J. Bone Joint Surg. 54-A:1408–1418, 1972.

Eaton, R. G., and Green, W. T.: Epimysiotomy and fasciotomy in the treatment of Volkmann's ischemic contracture. Orthop. Clin. North Am. 3:175–185, 1972.

Eaton, R. G., and Green, W. T.: Volkmann's ischemia. A volar compartment syndrome of the forearm. Clin. Orthop. 113:58–64, 1975.

Eichler, G. R., and Lipscomb, P. R.: The changing treatment of Volkmann's ischemic contractures from 1955 to 1965 at the Mayo Clinic. Clin. Orthop. 50:215–223, 1967.

Eiken, O., Nabseth, D. C., Mayer, R. F., and Deterling, R. A.: Limb replantation. Arch. Surg. 88:70–75, 1964.

Elliott, M. J., and Glass, K. D.: Anterior tibial compartment syndrome associated with ergotamine ingestion. Clin. Orthop. 118:44–47, 1976.

Ellis, H.: Disabilities after tibial shaft fractures, with special reference to Volkmann's ischaemic contracture. J. Bone Joint Surg. 40-B:190–197, 1958.

Flynn, J. C., Matthews, J. G., and Benoit, R. L.: Blind pinning of displaced supracondylar fractures of the humerus in children. J. Bone Joint Surg. 56-A:263–272, 1974.

Fowler, P. J., and Willis, R. B.: Vascular compartment syndromes. Can. J. Surg. 18:157–161, 1975.

Franz, D. R., Berberich, J. J., Blake, S., and Mills, W. J., Jr.: Evaluation of fasciotomy and vasodilator for treatment of frostbite in the dog. Cryobiology 15:659–669, 1978.

Freedman, B. J., and Knowles, C. H. R.: Anterior tibial syndrome due to arterial embolism and thrombosis. Br. Med. J. 1:270, 1959.

Garfin, S. R., Castilonia, R. R., Mubarak, S. J., Hargens, A. R., Akeson, W. H., and Russell, F. E.: Role of surgical decompression in treatment of rattlesnake bites. Surg. Forum 30:502–504, 1979A.

Garfin, S. R., Mubarak, S. J., and Davidson, T. M.: Rattlesnake bites: current concepts. Clin. Orthop. 140:50–57, 1979B.

Gelberman, R. H., Garfin, S. R., Hergenroeder, P. T., Mubarak, S. J., and Menon, J.: Compartment syndromes of the forearm: diagnosis and treatment. Clin. Orthop., 1981, in press.

Gitlitz, G. F.: The anterior tibial compartment syndrome. A complication of a femoropopliteal bypass procedure. Vasc. Dis 2:122–130, 1965.

Glass, T. G.: Early debridement in pit viper bites. J.A.M.A. 235:2513, 1976.

Goodfellow, J., Fearn, B. D'A., and Mathews, J. M.: Iliacus haematoma: a common complication of haemophilia. J. Bone Joint Surg. 49-B:748–756, 1967.

Grace, T. G., Campbell, E. L., and Omer, G. E.: Management of venomous wounds. Orthop. Trans. 2:254–255, 1978.

Griffiths, D. L.: Volkmann's ischaemic contracture. Br. J. Surg. 28:239–260, 1940.

Grosz, C. R., Shafton, G. W., Kottmeier, P. K., and Herbsman, H.: Volkmann's contracture and femoral shaft fractures. J. Trauma 13:129–131, 1973.

Halpern, A. A., Mochizuki, R., and Long, C. E.: Compartment syndrome of the forearm following radial artery puncture in a patient treatment with anticoagulants. J. Bone Joint Surg. 60-A:1136–1137, 1978.

Halpern, A. A., and Nagel, D. A.: Bilateral compartment syndrome associated with androgen therapy. Clin. Orthop. 128:243–246, 1977.

Harrison, R., and Jackson, P. E.: Anterior tibial syndrome after acute arterial occlusion, treated by decompression. Br. Med. J. 1:403, 1956.

Hawkins, L. G., Lischer, C. G., and Sweeney, M.: The main line accidental intra-arterial drug injection. A review of seven cases. Clin. Orthop. 94:268–274, 1973.

Henderson, B., and Dujon, E.: Snake bites in children. J. Pediatr. Surg. 8:729, 1973.

Hey Groves, E. W.: A clinical lecture upon the surgical aspects of haemophilia with special reference to two cases of Volkmann's contracture resulting from this disease. Br. Med. J. 1:611–614, 1907.

Hill, R. L., and Brookes, B.: Volkmann's ischemic contracture in hemophilia. Am. Surg. 103:444–449, 1936.

Holden, C. E. A.: Compartmental syndromes following trauma. Clin. Orthop. 113:95–102, 1975.

Horn, J. S., and Sevitt, S.: Ischaemic necrosis and regeneration of the tibialis anterior muscle after rupture of the popliteal artery. J. Bone Joint Surg. 33-B:348–358, 1951.

Huang, T. T., Lynch, J. B., Larson, D. L., and Lewis, S. R.: The use of excisional therapy in the management of snakebite. Ann. Surg. 179:598, 1974.

Hughes, J. R.: Ischaemic necrosis of the anterior muscle due to fatigue. J. Bone Joint Surg. 30-B:581–594, 1948.

Jackson, J. P., and Waugh, W.: The technique and complications of upper tibial osteotomy; a review of 226 operations. J. Bone Joint Surg. 56-B:236–245, 1974.

Jacob, J. E.: Compartment syndrome. Int. Surg. 59:542–548, 1974.

Jepson, P. N.: Ischemic contracture. Experimental study. Am. Surg. 84:785–795, 1926.

Justis, D. L., Law, E. J., and MacMillan, B. G.: Tibial compartment syndromes in burn patients. A report of four cases. Arch. Surg. 111:1004–1008, 1976.

Kelly, G. L., and Eiseman, B.: Civilian vascular injuries. J. Trauma 15:507–514, 1975.

Kunkel, M. G., and Lynn, R. B.: The anterior tibial compartment syndrome. Can. J. Surg. 1:212–217, 1958.

Küttner, H., and Baruch, M.: Beitr. Klin. Chir. 1:120, 1920.

Lancourt, J. E., Gilbert, M. S., and Posner, M. A.: Management of bleeding and associated complications of hemophilia in the hand and forearm. J. Bone Joint Surg. 59-A:451–460, 1977.

Leach, R. E., Hammond, G., and Stryker, W. S.: Anterior tibial compartment syndrome: acute and chronic. J. Bone Joint Surg. 49-A:451–462, 1967.

Lees, A. J.: Anterior tibial compartment syndrome following prolonged tetany. J. Neurol. Psychiatry 39:406–408, 1976.

Leriche, R.: Surgery of the sympathetic system. Indications and results. Ann. Surg. 88:449–469, 1928.

Lipscomb, L. R.: The etiology and prevention of Volkmann's ischemic contracture. Surg. Gynecol. Obstet. 103:353–361, 1956.

Luce, E. A., Futrell, J. W., Wilgis, E. F. S., and Hoopes, J. E.: Compression neuropathy following brachial arterial puncture in anticoagulated patients. J. Trauma 16:717–721, 1976.

Lytton, B., and Blandy, J. P.: Anterior tibial syndrome after embolectomy. Br. J. Surg. 48:346–348, 1960.

Mann, R. J., and Wallquist, J. M.: Early decompression fasciotomy in the treatment of high voltage electrical burns of the extremities. South Med. J. 68:1103–1108, 1975.

Manson, I. W.: Post partum eclampsia complicated by the anterior tibial syndrome. Br. Med. J. 2:1117–1118, 1964.

Maor, P., Levy, M., Lotem, M., and Fried, A.: Iatrogenic Volkmann's ischemia: a result of pressure-transfusion. Int. Surg. 57:415–416, 1972.

Matsen, F. A., III: Compartmental syndrome: a unified concept. Clin. Orthop. 113:8–13, 1975.

Matsen, F. A., and Staheli, L. T.: Neurovascular complications following tibial osteotomy in children. A case report. Clin. Orthop. 110:210–214, 1975.

Moncrief, J. A.: Burns. In Schwartz, S. I. (ed.): Principles of Surgery. McGraw-Hill Book Co., New York, 1969.

Montgomery, A. H., and Ireland, J.: Traumatic segmentary arterial spasm. J.A.M.A. 105:1741–1746, 1935.

Morgan, N. R., Waugh, T. R., and Boback, M. D.: Volkmann's ischemic contracture after intra-arterial injection of secobarbital. J.A.M.A. 212:476–478, 1970.

Mozes, M., Ramon, Y., and Jahr, T.: The anterior tibial syndrome. Bone Joint Surg. 44-A:730, 1962.

Mubarak, S. J., and Carroll, N. C.: Volkmann's contracture in children: Aetiology and prevention. J. Bone Joint Surg. 61-B:285–293, 1979.

Mustard, W. T., and Simmons, E. H.: Experimental arterial spasm in the lower extremities produced by traction. J. Bone Joint Surg. 35-B:437–441, 1953.

Neviaser, R. J., Adams, J. P., and May, G. I.: Complications of arterial puncture in anticoagulated patients. J. Bone Joint Surg. 58-A:218–220, 1976.

Nicholson, J. T., Foster, R. M., and Heath, R. D.: Bryant's traction: a provocative cause of circulatory complications. J.A.M.A. 157:415–418, 1955.

Owen, R., and Tsimboukis, B.: Ischaemia complicating closed tibial and fibular shaft fractures. J. Bone Joint Surg. 49-B:268–275, 1967.

Patman, R. D.: Compartmental syndromes in peripheral vascular surgery. Clin. Orthop. 113:103–110, 1975.

Patman, R. D., and Thompson, J. E.: Fasciotomy in peripheral vascular surgery. Arch. Surg. 101:663–670, 1970.

Paton, D. F.: The pathogenesis of anterior tibial syndrome. J. Bone Joint Surg. 50-B:383–385, 1968.

Pruitt, B. A., Jr., Dowling, J. A., and Moncrief, J. A.: Escharotomy in early burn care. Arch. Surg. 96:502–507, 1968.

Rich, N. M., Manion, W. C., and Hughes, C. W.: Surgical and pathological evaluation of vascular injuries in Vietnam. J. Trauma 9:279–291, 1969.

Rorabeck, C. H., and MacNab, I.: The anterior tibial compartment syndrome complicating fractures of the shaft of the tibia. J. Bone Joint Surg. 58-A:549–550, 1976.

Rosengart, R., Nelson, R. J., and Emmanoulides, G. C.: Anterior tibial compartment syndrome in a child: an unusual complication of cardiac catheterization. Pediatrics 58:456–458, 1976.

Russell, F. E., Carson, R. W., Wainschel, J., and Osborne, A. H.: Snake venom poisoning in the United States: experience with 550 cases. J.A.M.A. 233:341, 1975.

Salisbury, R. E., McKeel, D. W., and Mason, A. D.: Ischemic necrosis of the intrinsic muscles of the hand after thermal injuries. J. Bone Joint Surg. 56-A:1701–1707, 1974.

Schrock, R. D.: Peroneal nerve palsy following derotation osteotomies for tibial torsion. Clin. Orthop. 62:172–177, 1969.

Scott, W. H., Jacobs, B., and Lockshin, M. D.: Posterior compartment syndrome resulting from a dissecting popliteal cyst. Clin. Orthop. 122:189–192, 1977.

Sheridan, G. W., and Matsen, F. A.: Fasciotomy in the treatment of the acute compartment syndrome. J. Bone Joint Surg. 58-A:112–115, 1976.

Sirbu, A. B., Murphy, M. J., and White, A. S.: Soft tissue complications of fracture of the leg. Calif. West. Med. 60:53–56, 1944.

Steel H. H., Sandrow, R. E., and Sullivan, P. D.: Complications of tibial osteotomy in children for genu varum or valgum. J. Bone Joint Surg. 53-A:1629–1635, 1971.

Stone, H. H., Cantwell, D. V., and Fulenwider, J. T.: Wringer arm injuries. J. Pediatr. Surg. 11:375–379, 1976.

Suffee, J., Zeluff, G. R., and Warden, G. D.: Natural history of intramuscular pressure following thermal injury to the upper extremities. American Burn Association, New Orleans, Mar. 13, 1979.

Sweeney, H. E., and O'Brien, G. F.: Bilateral anterior tibial syndrome in association with the nephrotic syndrome: report of a case. Arch. Intern. Med. 116:487–490, 1965.

Thomas, H. B.: Some orthopaedic findings in ninety-eight cases of haemophilia. J. Boint Joint Surg. 18:140–147, 1936.

Thomson, S. A., and Mahoney, L. J.: Volkmann's ischaemic contracture and its relationship to fracture of the femur. J. Bone Joint Surg. 33-B:336–347, 1951.

Tilney, N. L., and McLamb, J. R.: Leg trauma with posterior tibial artery tear. J. Trauma 7:807–810, 1967.

Wall, J. J.: Compartment syndrome as a complication of the Hauser procedure. J. Bone Joint Surg. 61-A:185–191, 1979.

Watson, D. C.: Anterior tibial syndrome following arterial embolism. Br. Med. J. 1:1412–1414, 1955.

Weitz, E. M., and Carson, G.: The anterior tibial compartment syndrome in a twenty month old infant. A complication of the use of a bow leg brace. Bull. Hosp. Joint Dis. 30:16–20, 1969.

Wells, J., and Templeton, J.: Femoral neuropathy associated with anticoagulant therapy. Clin. Orthop. 124:155–160, 1977.

Whitesides, T. E., Jr., Hirada, H., and Morimoto, K.: Compartment syndromes and the role of fasciotomy, its parameters and techniques. Am. Acad. Orthop. Surg. Instructional Course Lectures 26:179–194, 1977.

Wiggins, H. E.: The anterior tibial compartmental syndrome. A complication of the Hauser procedure. Clin. Orthop. 113:90–94, 1975.

Winslow, P. M.: Circulatory complications from Bryant's traction. Read before Inter-urban Orthopaedic Club Program, Rochester, New York, Oct. 19, 1950.

Wolfort, F. G., Mogelvang, L. C., and Filtzer, H. S.: Anterior tibial compartment syndrome following muscle hernia repair. Arch. Surg. 106:97–99, 1973.

Chapter Six

CLINICAL DIAGNOSIS OF ACUTE COMPARTMENT SYNDROMES

Charles A. Owen, M.D.

The early diagnosis of compartment syndromes depends on recognition of the clinical signs and symptoms of increased intracompartmental pressure. In many cases, pressure measurement is not necessary but may be only confirmatory. In others, however, clinical findings are confusing and the diagnosis may depend almost entirely on intracompartmental pressure measurements. The purpose of this chapter is to discuss the typical signs and symptoms, with emphasis on the deficiency of the clinical examination in some situations (Fig. 6–1).

HISTORY

Early authors were concerned primarily with the pathogenesis of Volkmann's ischemic contracture, and made little mention of the clinical findings in the acute phase. Murphy (1914) and Jepson (1926) did describe the classic acute findings, but until their concept of treatment by decompressive fasciotomy was well accepted there was little reason for accurate early diagnosis. In his influential Hunterian lecture and article, Griffiths (1940) confused the separate, but sometimes concomitant, entities of major vascular insufficiency and compartment syndrome. Out of this confusion grew the mnemonic four P's of Volkmann's ischemic contracture: "pain, pallor, paralysis, and pulselessness" (Griffiths, 1940, 1948). Despite the appearance of many articles over the following 30 years pointing out that indications of distal ischemia such as pallor and pulselessness are not signs of compartment syndrome, this mnemonic persists.

98

SIGNS AND SYMPTOMS

Pain

The first and most important symptom of an impending compartment syndrome is pain that is greater than that expected from the primary problem, e.g., the fracture or contusion. The pain is usually described as a deep, throbbing feeling of pressure that is unrelenting. It is localized to the segment of the limb containing the affected compartment, and not referred into the distribution of the traversing sensory nerves, since nerve ischemia ordinarily produces failure of function without pain. The pain is not relieved by immobilization, and indeed may be aggravated by the use of a rigid circumferential dressing such as a cast.

Many authors comment on the occasional lack of pain as a presenting symptom but, in our experience, absence of pain is almost always due to a superimposed central or peripheral sensory deficit. In the drug overdose-limb compression syndrome, patients are often comatose or obtunded. A concomitant injury to a peripheral nerve may also eliminate pain as a presenting symptom. For example, a compartment syndrome developing after arterial reconstruction of a lacerated axillary artery would not produce pain if the brachial plexus had been lacerated simultaneously.

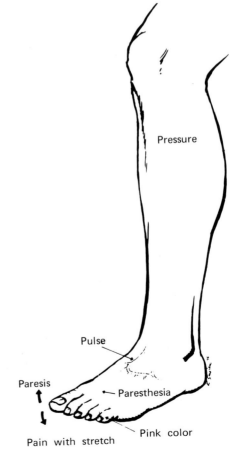

Figure 6–1 Early findings of a compartment syndrome with anterior tibial compartment involvement. Of these six P's, increased pressure is the earliest finding. (With permission from Mubarak, S. J., et al.: Laboratory diagnosis of orthopedic diseases: muscle pressure measurement with the wick catheter. *In* Practice of Surgery. Harper & Row, New York, 1978, Chap. 20, pp. 1–8.

In most patients, however, pain remains the first and most important symptom. We have studied intracompartmental pressures in the immediate postoperative period in several patients placed in a cylinder cast following a high tibial osteotomy. The appearance of pain as a symptom quite clearly correlated with increasing intracompartmental pressure. Pain became severe as pressures approached 30 mm Hg (Fig. 8–6).

Tense Compartment

The earliest and only truly objective finding is a swollen, palpably tense compartment that is a direct manifestation of increased intracompartmental pressure. The tenseness is not localized to the area of injury, e.g., the fracture or contusion. Increased pressure equilibrates rapidly throughout the compartment, producing perceptible tenseness in all areas of the compartment. The overlying skin is sometimes shiny and warm, this and the palpable tenderness all give an impression of cellulitis.

Dressings and casts frequently cover the involved compartment(s) and prevent examination by palpation and inspection. Obviously, all dressing should be removed to allow adequate examination of the limb; casts should be univalved and spread, bivalved, or removed. Concern over loss of fracture reduction should not cause procrastination in removing sufficient plaster to allow adequate examination. Removal of constrictive dressings or casts is also important as a first step in treatment of an impending compartment syndrome.

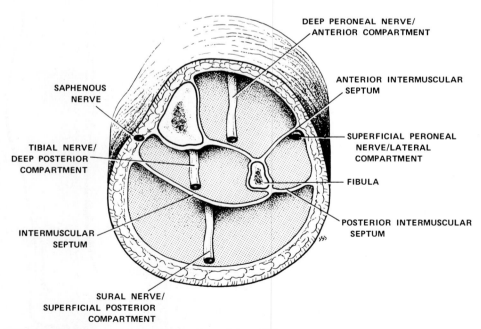

Figure 6–2 Cross-section at the junction of the middle and distal thirds of the leg, illustrating the four compartments and their respective nerves. (With permission from Mubarak, S. J., and Owen, C. A.: Double-incision fasciotomy of the leg for decompression in compartment syndromes. J. Bone Joint Surg. 59-A:184–187, 1977.)

Although it is not possible, even with experience, to consistently estimate by palpation the degree to which intracompartmental pressures are elevated, the presence of significant tenseness throughout the compartment boundaries suggests an impending or established compartment syndrome. Conversely, if there are areas of the compartment that are palpably soft, the examiner may be reassured that for the moment, at least, compartment pressures are not elevated.

The most difficult compartment to evaluate by palpation is the deep posterior of the leg, because it is buried under the superficial posterior compartment. This may account for the apparent frequency with which the diagnosis is missed in this compartment (Seddon, 1966).

Pain with Muscle Stretch

Pain with passive stretch of the muscles in the involved compartment is a common finding, usually attributed to muscle ischemia. Stretch pain is not, however, a specific sign of a compartment syndrome. If the underlying problem has caused direct muscle injury, such as in a contusion or fracture, passive stretch of this injured muscle will in itself produce pain. Furthermore, children commonly exhibit pain with passive stretch of the finger flexors following forearm and elbow injuries, even in the absence of significantly elevated intracompartmental pressure. Patients with sensory deficits, either central or peripheral, may not exhibit stretch pain, even in the presence of elevated intracompartmental pressure.

Sensory Deficit

Most compartments are traversed by nerves having distal sensory distribution (Fig. 6–2). The first sign of nerve ischemia is the alteration of sensation, manifested early by subjective paresthesias in the distribution of the involved nerve, followed by hypoesthesia and later anesthesia. We have documented the appearance of paresthesias in the distribution of the deep peroneal nerve with anterior compartment pressure greater than 30 mm Hg.

With only a few exceptions, all our patients with intracompartmental pressure over 30 mm Hg have exhibited sensory deficit. We consider, therefore, that unless there is superimposed central or peripheral nerve deficit, decreased sensation to light touch or pinprick in the distal sensory distribution is a very reliable sign of increased intracompartmental pressure. Furthermore, the specific nerve involvement is indicative of which compartment(s) are involved. In the leg, for example, first web space involvement (deep peroneal) implicates the anterior compartment; dorsum of foot (superficial peroneal), the lateral; lateral foot (sural), the superficial posterior; sole of the foot (posterior tibial), the deep posterior compartment.

Motor Weakness

Paresis secondary to nerve or neuromuscular junction ischemia and elevated intracompartmental pressure is a relatively late physical finding. The clinical experience of many authors documents a sequence of nerve deficit from paresthesia to sensory loss, to motor weakness, to paralysis. This correlates well with the experimental evidence of Hargens et al. (1979), who demonstrated that the large, fast-conducting fibers are selectively blocked at lower intracompartmental pressures than are the smaller, slower-conducting fibers.

Paresis may be confusing, however, because it may be secondary to a proximal nerve injury rather than intracompartmental ischemia. Likewise, guarding because of pain may prevent a full voluntary contraction, simulating paresis.

It should be emphasized that motor weakness that is clearly related to increased intracompartmental pressure, although often confusing, is a late sign and an indication for prompt action.

Pulses

Impairment of circulation distal to the involved compartment, as manifested by absence of pulses, decreased capillary fill, or pallor, has long been associated with Volkmann's ischemic contracture. As previously noted, the Griffiths (1948) mnemonic has perpetuated the misconception that distal circulation is frequently impaired by increased intracompartmental pressures.

Although intracompartmental pressures of 30 to 60 mm Hg can produce ischemia of muscle and nerve within the compartment, such pressures are insufficient to occlude flow through a major artery having a much higher intraluminal pressure (Fig. 6–3). For example, although a pressure of 50 mm Hg in the anterior tibial compartment could cause ischemia and necrosis of the muscles and nerves within the compartment, such a pressure would be insufficient to shut down the anterior tibial artery traversing the compartment, and the dorsalis pedis pulse would, therefore, be intact. It should be obvious that, in the normotensive patient, only the extremely rare intracompartmental pressure approaching 100 mm Hg could hydrodynamically occlude distal pulses. Matsen et al. (1977) recorded an intact dorsalis pedis pulse in human volunteers with elevation of the anterior compartmental pressure to as high as 80 mm Hg by means of a segmental cylindric air splint.

It has been suggested that absent pulses may result from vascular spasm secondary to elevated intracompartmental pressures. Eaton and Green (1975) state that it was possible experimentally to produce transient complete spasm of the brachial artery in the rabbit injecting a small bolus of autogenous blood beneath the volar carpal ligament. In our own laboratory, however, pressurization of the entire anterolateral compartment in a small number of dogs to as high as 80 mm Hg produced only very occasional and very transient spasm in middle-sized vessels, as seen on angiography. No occlusion of the major vessels by spasm was noted. It is our opinion that spasm secondary to elevated intracompartmental pressures as a cause of persistently absent pulses and distal ischemia is distinctly unusual.

Except in the presence of major arterial injury or disease, peripheral pulses and capillary filling are routinely intact in compartment syndrome patients. Although intracompartmental pressure is high enough to cause ischemia of muscle and nerve by occluding microcirculation within the compartment, it only very rarely is high enough to occlude the major arteries. If peripheral pulses are absent, other causes for major arterial obstruction must be sought. Arteriography is indicated.

Conversely, the presence of distal pulses and capillary fill is no reassurance that

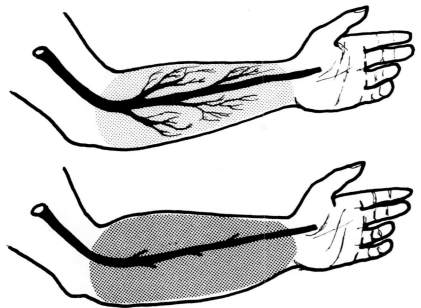

Figure 6–3 Schematic of forearm compartment syndrome. Intracompartmental pressures are only rarely high enough to occlude the major arteries of the compartment. However, the pressure is sufficient to cause ischemia of muscle and nerve by occluding the microcirculation within the compartment. (With permission from Rang, M.: Children's Fractures. J. B. Lippincott Co., Philadelphia, 1974.)

a compartment syndrome does not exist. Failure to appreciate this fact may lead to a false sense of security and a failure to institute prompt treatment for the increased intracompartmental pressure.

DIFFERENTIAL DIAGNOSIS

Many of the underlying etiologies precipitating compartment syndromes in themselves produce a painful, swollen extremity. The diagnosis of the underlying problem, e.g., fracture or contusion, is obvious; the diagnosis of a superimposed compartment syndrome is more difficult. Conditions such as cellulitis, osteomyelitis, stress fracture, tenosynovitis, and deep vein thrombosis may result in painful swelling in the extremities, but rarely, if ever, do they cause compartment syndromes. In cellulitis, the signs and symptoms of infection are present. Acute compartment syndromes do not produce significant leukocytosis or fever unless secondary infection develops. Stress fracture causes little swelling and no palpable compartmental tenseness. Tenderness usually is well localized over the fracture. The problem of differential diagnosis in the chronic compartment syndrome is discussed in Chapter 14. Deep vein thrombosis may produce calf swelling, palpable tenseness, and stretch pain. The differential diagnosis between this and a superficial or deep posterior compartment syndrome may be difficult, requiring venography and pressure studies.

The most complex differential diagnoses arise in distinguishing compartment syndrome, arterial occlusion, and neurapraxia. These conditions frequently coexist,

Table 6-1 TYPICAL CLINICAL FINDINGS OF COMPARTMENT
SYNDROME, ARTERIAL OCCLUSION, AND NEURAPRAXIA*

	Compartment Syndrome	Arterial Occlusion	Neurapraxia
Pressure increased in compartment	+	−	−
Pain with stretch	+	+	−
Paresthesia or anesthesia	+	+	+
Paresis or paralysis	+	+	+
Pulses intact	+	−	+

*With permission from Mubarak, S., and Carroll, N.: Volkmann's contracture in children: aetiology and prevention. J. Bone Joint Surg. 61-B:290, 1979.

and their clinical findings often overlap, making diagnosis difficult, if not impossible (Table 6–1). All may have associated motor or sensory deficit and pain. The arterial injury usually results in absent pulses, poor skin color, and decreased skin temperature. In contrast, the compartment syndrome routinely presents with intact peripheral circulation, unless the underlying etiology is arterial injury or disease. Nerve injuries usually give little pain, and the diagnosis is often by exclusion of the other two entities. Doppler, arteriography, and pressure measurements are frequently required to aid in the differential diagnosis of these three conditions.

DEFICIENCIES OF CLINICAL SIGNS AND SYMPTOMS

The clinical diagnosis of compartment syndrome is frequently confusing because of the lack of truly objective findings. The evaluation of the severity of pain is obviously difficult, and errors are made in both directions. Hyperreactive patients may complain bitterly with minimal pain, whereas stoic individuals may not complain even with significantly elevated intracompartmental pressures. Palpable compartmental tenseness remains the only true objective finding, and at best is only a rough indicator of intracompartmental pressure. The other signs of muscle stretch pain, sensory deficit, and motor strength all depend on patient cooperation and response.

In our prospective analysis of suspected compartment syndromes, we identified three groups of patients in whom difficulties in eliciting or interpreting the physical findings are frequently encountered and measurement of intracompartmental pressure is extremely helpful (Mubarak et al., 1978):

Uncooperative or Unreliable Patients. Children with elbow or forearm fracture, for example, may be so frightened that a careful motor and sensory evaluation is not possible. Movement of their fingers may be followed by painful cries that defy accurate interpretation. In the adult, alcohol and other drugs may make interpretation of clinical signs difficult or impossible.

Unresponsive Patients. The patient with drug overdose-limb compression syndrome is commonly obtunded or comatose on admission, or may be on a respirator. The only reliable physical finding may be a swollen extremity.

Patients with Peripheral Nerve Deficit Attributable to Other Etiologies. It is often hard to differentiate neurapraxia secondary to stretch or contusion of a nerve from neurologic deficits resulting from increased intracompartmental pressures. We see this problem most commonly in patients with proximal leg injuries and peroneal nerve deficits. The importance of differentiation is obvious, since the neurapraxia group almost uniformly recover without treatment, whereas those having compartment syndromes require fasciotomy.

Similarly, in patients with known proximal nerve deficits, such as laceration of brachial plexus, the neurologic examination is of no value in the diagnosis of a suspected concomitant compartment syndrome.

In summary, although we believe that the diagnosis of compartment syndrome can often be made clinically, we recommend the use of intracompartmental pressure measurements whenever clinical signs and symptoms are absent or confusing.

REFERENCES

Eaton, R. G., and Green, W. T.: Volkmann's ischemia. A volar compartment syndrome of the forearm. Clin. Orthop. 113:58–64, 1975.

Griffiths, D. L.: Volkmann's ischaemic contracture. Br. J. Surg. 28:239, 1940.

Griffiths, D. L.: The management of acute circulatory failure in an injured limb. J. Bone Joint Surg. 30-B:280–298, 1948.

Hargens, A. R., Romine, J. S., Sipe, J. C., Evans, K. L., Mubarak, S. J., and Akeson, W. H.: Peripheral nerve-conduction block by high muscle compartment pressure. J. Bone Surg. 61-A:192–200, 1979.

Jepson, P. N.: Ischemic contracture. Experimental study. Ann. Surg. 84:785, 1926.

Matsen, F. A., III, Mayo, K. A., Krugmire, R. B. J., Sheridan, G. W., and Kroft, G. H.: A model compartment syndrome in man with particular reference to the quantification of nerve function. J. Bone Joint Surg. 59-A:648–653, 1977.

Mubarak, S. J., Owen, C. A., Hargens, A. R., Garetto, L. P., and Akeson, W. H.: Acute compartment syndromes: diagnosis and treatment with the aid of the wick catheter. J. Bone Joint Surg. 60-A:1091–1095, 1978.

Murphy, J. B.: Myositis. J.A.M.A. 63:1249, 1914.

Seddon, H. J.: Volkmann's ischaemia in the lower limb. J. Bone Joint Surg. 48-B:627–636, 1966.

Chapter Seven

LABORATORY DIAGNOSIS OF ACUTE COMPARTMENT SYNDROMES

Alan R. Hargens, Ph.D.
and Scott J. Mubarak, M.D.

INTRODUCTION

As emphasized in Chapters 1 and 4, which cover the definition and pathophysiology of a compartment syndrome, high tissue fluid pressure is the pathogenic factor that is common to all acute compartment syndromes. Owing to confinement of skeletal muscle within relatively tight, fascial containers, any increase in intracompartmental volume following trauma or postischemic swelling produces high intracompartmental pressure. This, in turn, reduces capillary blood flow to a level that jeopardizes viability of intracompartmental tissues. Within a period of a few hours, a sequence of pain, neurologic deficit, and intracompartmental necrosis will result if the vicious cycle of "elevated intracompartmental pressure–tissue ischemia" is not interrupted by prompt decompression. Thus, it is obvious that measurement of intracompartmental pressure is probably the most objective and reliable parameter for laboratory diagnosis of acute compartment syndromes.

Indications for intracompartmental pressure measurement exist when a possible compartment syndrome is being diagnosed in patients who are comatose, unresponsive, or uncooperative (e.g., a frightened child), and also in cases of primary neurapraxia versus acute compartment syndrome. Pressure measurements are helpful but less critical when clinical documentation is complete, when verifying the adequacy of decompression during fasciotomy, or when monitoring skin closure.

Since tissue fluid pressure is important in terms of compartment syndrome pathogenesis and diagnosis, this chapter emphasizes clinical measurements of intracompartmental pressure and their significance. However, before this procedure is fully detailed, a brief history of techniques for monitoring tissue pressure is presented, and modern clinical methods and equipment are critically evaluated. Our section on intracompartmental pressure measurement ends with a threshold pressure at which decompressive fasciotomy is recommended based on past clinical and animal studies of tissue necrosis related to pressure-time variables.

Finally, other laboratory criteria that aid the diagnosis of acute compartment syndromes are discussed. These include blood and urine tests, electromyography, nerve function studies, and assessments of peripheral circulation.

MEASUREMENT OF INTRACOMPARTMENTAL PRESSURE

Historical Background

NEEDLE TECHNIQUES

The first direct attempts at measuring tissue fluid pressure, also called interstitial fluid pressure (P_t), were made by subcutaneous needle cannulations (Landerer, 1884). This technique involved inserting a fine needle into the tissues and measuring the hydrostatic pressure required to inject a saline solution. This study was followed by several others (Burch and Sodeman, 1937; Wells et al., 1938; McMaster, 1946) that refined the method to minute injection volumes. These measurements, performed mostly in mammals, yielded pressures in a range from 0 to +10 mm Hg.

The needle puncture technique, however, has several critical liabilities. First, most of the investigations before 1940 involved the injection of relatively large amounts (0.1 $mm^3 \cdot min^{-1}$ to 0.5 $mm^3 \cdot min^{-1}$) of saline into the tissue, thus producing local edema. Even McMaster (1946) noted slight edematous conditions when 0.06 $mm^3 \cdot 5\ min^{-1}$ was infused. Furthermore, if the tissues had negative P_t, a saline solution injected by needle enters spontaneously until ambient pressure is reached. Therefore, to attempt a measurement of P_t by additional infusion of saline (continuing the distention of the interstitial spaces) exaggerates the edema and positive P_t further. Such a technique exhibits a direct correlation between the amount of infusion and the level of positive P_t. Comparing the P_t values with infusion volumes, McMaster (1946) indeed found such a correlation. Second, since the minute interstitial spaces have a high resistance to flow and since these needles have a very small pick-up area, needle puncture measurements are particularly susceptible to conditions of localized tissue trauma (especially the extraneous conditions caused by the probe insertion) and tissue compliance.

Measurements of intracompartmental pressure by saline injection through needles were first applied to diagnosis of chronic compartment syndromes by French and Price (1962) and Reneman (1968), and diagnosis of acute compartment syndromes by Whitesides and co-workers (1975A, B). Later, Matsen and associates (1976) used a variation of the needle technique that employs continuous infusion of saline (McMaster, 1946) to aid diagnosis of compartment syndromes.

A further refinement of the needle technique was developed by Wiederhielm (1968) using a micropuncture technique described earlier (Wiederhielm et al., 1964). Wiederhielm (1969) has found positive interstitial fluid pressures averaging + 2.2 cm H_2O in the free-fluid spaces of bat wings. This technique consists of 0.1 to 1 μm glass micropipettes placed in the free-fluid spaces. The micropipettes are filled with

1 to 2 M NaCl, necessary to facilitate electronic measurements of hydrostatic pressure. Micropipettes are usually broken when inserted through skin, so this technique is not applicable to diagnosis of compartment syndromes in humans.

CHRONICALLY-IMPLANTED CAPSULE TECHNIQUE

Guyton (1963) was the first to measure negative (subambient) P_t in the interstitial spaces. In his pioneering studies Guyton implanted 200 spherical, perforated plastic capsules (1- to 2-cm diameter) subcutaneously in dogs. Three to four weeks after the chronic implantation, scar tissue had grown in through the perforations, forming a complete lining over the capsule's inner surface. When needles connected to pressure transducers were inserted into the free-fluid space within these capsules, a negative P_t averaging -6 mm Hg was recorded. Furthermore, Guyton's capsules closely followed capillary dynamics induced by tissue dehydration, tissue hydration, and changes in arterial and venous pressure (Guyton, 1963). It has been suggested, however, that these capsules excluded some proteins and glycosaminoglycans, and thus there was a colloid osmotic pressure effect in addition to the P_t effect operating through the capsule (Stromberg and Wiederhielm, 1970). This would tend to make Guyton's P_t measurements slightly more negative than those actually present in the interstitial spaces. Refuting the argument of Stromberg and Wiederhielm, Guyton et al. (1971) found little impedance to protein movement into the capsules. Aside from the arguments for or against, the inescapable liability is that the capsule must be chronically implanted four to five weeks before making pressure measurements. Therefore, this technique is not applicable to a clinical diagnosis of acute compartment syndromes.

WICK CATHETER TECHNIQUE

Scholander and collaborators (1968) first developed a wick technique for acute measurements of P_t in subcutaneous, intramuscular, and peritoneal tissue spaces of animals (Fig. 7–1). Later, this technique was modified for clinical use (Mubarak et al., 1976, 1978A; Hargens et al., 1977A, B, 1979). The principal advantage of the wick catheter over needle techniques is that no injection or continuous infusion of saline is necessary to measure equilibrium P_t. Obviously any injection or infusion of saline will artificially raise P_t, especially in any tissue with a low edema compliance, such as muscle. The wick catheter was designed to prevent blockage of the catheter's tip by tissue and to maximize contact between saline in the catheter and fluids in the tissue. The cylindric wick fibers (10- to 20-μm diameter) afford a large fluid-pick-up area, and the saline-filled spaces between wick fibers have dimensions comparable to fluid spaces within tissue (0.1 to 1 μm). The wick catheter is moved several centimeters away from the point of insertion in order to minimize tissue disruption and irritation. Tissue fluid pressure P_t is measured immediately and continuously after insertion. There is no osmotic effect at the interstitial fluid-wick boundary, and even red cells freely penetrate the wick. Bleeding is easily detected, however, by a characteristic surge in positive pressure and a subsequent insensitivity in the wick's response to changes of P_t (probably due to coagulation of blood around the wick fibers). Wicks and wick catheters are also used to collect small volumes of tissue fluid for studies of transcapillary fluid exchange in animals

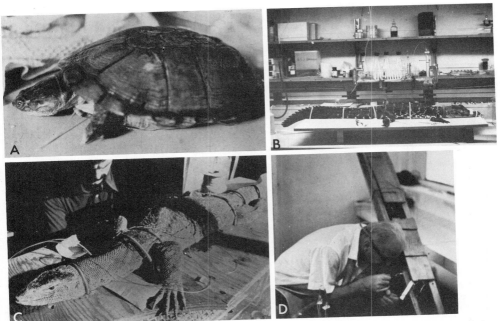

Figure 7-1 Examples of animal investigations of tissue fluid pressure with wick catheter technique (Scholander et al., 1968): *A*, Subcutaneous pressure measurement in the forelimb of a turtle; *B*, Tourniquet edema and pressure measurement in the forelimb of an alligator and in a lizard (*C*); and *D*, Dr. Scholander investigating the hydrostatic compensatory mechanism of a boa constrictor on a tilt table.

(Hargens et al., 1974; Fadnes and Aukland, 1977), trauma patients (Peters et al., 1981), and patients with early congestive heart failure (Noddeland et al., 1981).

SLIT CATHETER TECHNIQUE

The slit catheter, developed by Rorabeck et al. (1980) and later refined by Mubarak et al. (1981), combines advantages of several clinical techniques for measuring intracompartmental pressure. Five 3-mm long slits (approximately 60 degrees apart) in the tip of polyethylene tubing maintain continuity between tissue fluids and saline within the catheter without saline injection or flushing; this is an important feature in compartment syndromes in which P_t is already high and any increment of intracompartmental volume is contraindicated since transcapillary resorption is diminished or absent (Hargens et al., 1978). The slit catheter offers excellent response to changes of intramuscular pressure during muscle contraction by virtue of its large, multipetaled tip.

The reader may consult a more detailed review of interstitial fluid pressure (Guyton et al., 1971) and a recent compendium (Hargens, 1981) that together present an updated and complete review of tissue fluid pressure.

Comparison of Clinical Pressure Techniques

NEEDLE INJECTION TECHNIQUE

A needle injection technique (Whitesides et al., 1975A, B) commonly used for measuring intracompartmental pressure in compartment syndromes simply consists

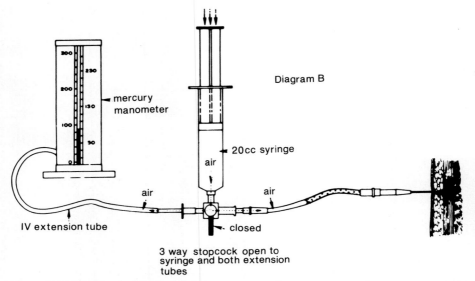

Figure 7–2 The needle injection technique measures intracompartmental pressure by raising air pressure until movement of saline into the tissue is detected via the saline-air meniscus. The air pressure at which saline is just injected is noted on the mercury manometer. (With permission from Whitesides et al., 1975A,B.)

of an 18-gauge needle connected to a 20-ml syringe by a saline and air column, which in turn is connected to a standard mercury manometer via a three-way stopcock (Fig. 7–2). Part of the extension tubing between the needle and the stopcock is filled with saline. After the needle is inserted into a given muscle compartment, air pressure within the syringe is raised until the saline-air meniscus just moves. Concurrently, this air pressure is measured on the mercury manometer.

The primary advantage of the needle injection technique is that all necessary equipment is simple, low-cost, and usually available in hospitals and offices. However, our experience and that of other investigators indicates that measurements by one physician or technician will often differ from those of another by 20 to 30 mm Hg, a degree of precision far below continuous infusion, wick catheter, and slit catheter techniques. Moreover, the needle injection method does not allow continuous monitoring of intracompartmental pressure, a feature desirable for determining: (1) the clinical course of an acute compartment syndrome; (2) the adequacy of decompression; or (3) the pressure during muscular contraction. With many hours of practice and careful attention to uniformity of procedure, precision to within ±5 mm Hg may be possible in the case of an experienced technician. Saline injection, however, overestimates intracompartmental pressures (Mubarak et al., 1976; Hargens et al., 1977B). In summary, we believe this technique should be used only as a last resort when other, more accurate equipment is not available.

CONTINUOUS INFUSION TECHNIQUE

Matsen and collaborators (1976, 1980, 1981) have developed a needle technique that allows continuous monitoring of intracompartmental pressure by a continuous, slow infusion of saline into the compartment at risk (Fig. 7–3). This technique probably represents the best means of long-term monitoring of compartmental pressure (up to three days, Matsen et al., 1981). Catheter tip coagulation and plugging is rarely a problem because of the infusion. Although this infusion technique allows continuous monitoring of intracompartmental pressure, measured pressure depends on the resistance of a given tissue to the creation of a small pocket of saline at the needle's tip (Brace et al., 1975). Therefore, completely accurate recordings of tissue fluid pressure are possible only when tissue compliance is very high. Since tissue compliance is considerably reduced at intracompartmental pressures above 30 mm Hg (see Fig. 4–5), this procedure tends to overestimate pressure in direct proportion to the amount of intracompartmental tamponade. In general, however, the continuous infusion technique records pressures that are only a few millimeters of mercury higher than the wick or slit catheter techniques in the range of 10 to 40 mm Hg (Hargens, unpublished observations).

The principal disadvantage of the continuous infusion procedure relates to the extra equipment involved, namely, the syringe-type infusion pump. This precision delivery pump is an expensive item that is not necessary for the wick or slit catheter technique. Moreover, these syringe pumps usually have one or more controls that set the rate of infusion. Thus, a minor switch of one control will increase the infusion rate by a factor of 100. Although a saline infusion rate of only 0.7 ml/day is recommended (Matsen et al., 1980), the infusion pump may deliver more than 70 ml/day if the controls are inadvertently switched to the wrong setting. This could have disastrous results in a patient being evaluated for an acute compartment syndrome.

Another disadvantage of the infusion technique lies in the measurement of muscular contraction or the study of chronic (recurrent) compartment syndromes. The slower response time compared with that for the wick and slit techniques does not allow for accurate measurement of changes in intracompartmental pressure during muscle contraction (Mubarak, unpublished observations).

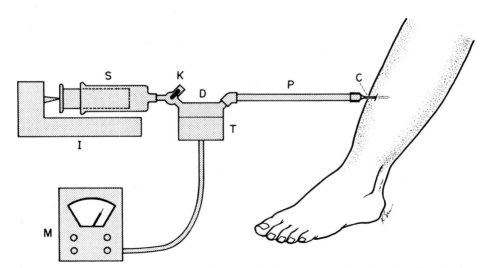

Figure 7–3 The continuous infusion technique maintains patency of needle tip by saline infusion at a rate of 0.7 ml/day. The technique employs three major pieces of equipment along with an 18- to 22-g needle and high pressure tubing. A syringe infusion pump (*I*) injects saline from a 3-ml syringe (*S*) through a three-way stopcock (*K*), pressure transducer dome (*D*), high pressure tubing (*P*), and finally through the needle catheter tip (*C*). The pressure at which this infusion occurs is measured by an arterial pressure transducer (*T*) and recorded on a standardized, amplification monitor (*M*). Continuous measurements of tissue resistance to saline infusion are obtained. (With permission from Matsen et al., 1980A.)

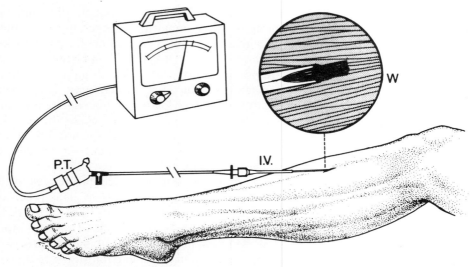

Figure 7–4 Wick catheter technique for measuring equilibrium, tissue fluid pressure continuously in a muscle compartment. An intravenous placement unit (*I.V.*) aids insertion of the sterilized saline-filled catheter. Before insertion, the wick catheter is connected to a pressure transducer (*P.T.*) and recorder, and calibrated. A close-up view of the catheter tip (*W*) illustrates how catheter patency and continuous fluid transmission are maintained by the numerous wick fibers. (With permission from Owen et al., N. Eng. J. Med. 300:1169–1172, 1979.)

Matsen and associates (1981) have suggested that a saline infusion technique is preferable to an equilibrium method such as the wick technique since the former (continuous infusion) measures "total tissue pressure" according to the Laplace law, whereas the latter (wick) measures "interstitial fluid pressure." However, the validity of such a separation of pressures is questionable (Wiederhielm, 1981), and moreover, Matsen and co-workers (1980, 1981) have found that the infusion technique measures pressures that are "virtually identical to those obtained from wick catheters" (1980).

WICK CATHETER TECHNIQUE

The clinical wick catheter (Mubarak et al., 1976; Hargens et al., 1977A, B, 1978, 1979) offers continuous equilibrium measurements of tissue fluid pressure without saline injection or infusion (Fig. 7–4). The accuracy and reproducibility of this technique have been verified in purely physical systems (Scholander et al., 1968) and in tissues (Mubarak et al., 1976; Hargens et al., 1978). The advantages of this method include a large area of tissue fluid pick-up by virtue of the wick fibers; maintenance of catheter patency without saline infusion (wick fibers maintain small channels of saline so that tissue does not plug the catheter's orifice); rapid attainment of equilibrium tissue fluid pressure; continuous monitoring of intracompartmental pressure even during contraction and exercise; and the ability to collect small samples of tissue fluid for other diagnostic procedures.

Disadvantages of the wick catheter include possible coagulation of blood around the catheter tip, which then requires some flushing to obtain good pressure response; possible hydrolysis of Dexon wick fibers during storage or prolonged tissue placement (Zeluff, 1978); and possible plugging of the catheter's tip during catheter manufacture as a result of using too much suture material. Another possible disadvantage of the wick catheter relates to loss of suture fibers in the tissue during removal of the catheter. However, during the past six years we have inserted over 800 catheters in human muscle and subcutaneous tissues without loss of wick materials and without the occurrence of any foreign-body reaction. With respect to the finding that Dexon wick fibers hydrolyze with time (Zeluff, 1978), we have since tested Dacron wick fibers and agree that these are better wick material than Dexon.

SLIT CATHETER TECHNIQUE

The slit catheter (Rorabeck et al., 1980) also combines long-term equilibrium measurements of intracompartmental pressure, ease of manufacture, and excellent response to muscle contraction without saline injection or infusion (Fig. 7–5). Although the slit catheter is relatively new and at present lacks some of the extensive clinical testing of other catheters, it combines several features that potentially make it ideal for measuring intracompartmental pressure in compartment syndromes. The manufacture of this catheter is theoretically more uniform and its use probably reduces the risk of leaving catheter materials behind after its removal. Slit catheters respond very well to changes in intracompartmental pressure, whether produced by palpation over the skin or by muscle contraction. Preliminary studies in our laboratory indicate that slit catheters are less prone to coagulation problems and that, when a clot forms around the catheter orifice, it is easily dislodged by applying finger pressure over the catheter tip. In this manner, catheter patency is maintained and good response is verified without any extraneous flushing or infusion of saline into the muscle compartment at risk (Mubarak et al., 1981).

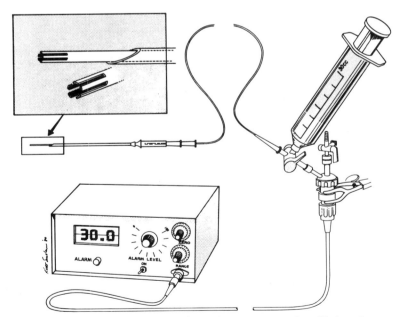

Figure 7–5 Slit catheter technique for continuous measurement of equilibrium, intracompartmental pressure. Prior to insertion into a muscle compartment, the sterile slit catheter is connected to the pressure transducer and digital recorder and then filled with saline via a 30-ml syringe. The catheter tip protrudes from the insertion needle during filling so that the tip can be checked for air bubbles (*see close-up, upper left*). Before insertion into muscle, the catheter is pulled entirely within the needle.

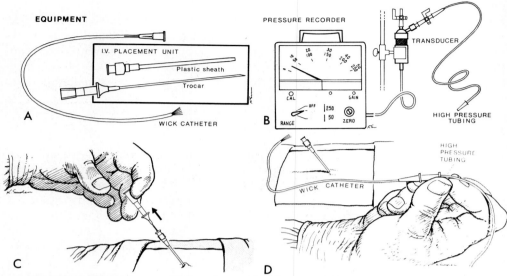

Figure 7–6 *A,* Equipment: Wick catheter, I.V. placement unit for insertion (inner steel trocar, plastic sheath). *B,* Set-up and preparation: Assistant sets up pressure recorder, transducer, high pressure tubing filled with sterile saline (the same equipment utilized for direct arterial blood pressure). Assistant may be anesthesiologist or a technician familiar with this equipment. *C,* Procedure: Under sterile conditions and local anesthesia, insert I.V. placement unit into muscle compartment to be studied and withdraw inner steel trocar. *D,* Connect wick catheter to high pressure tubing, fill with sterile saline, and flush out all air bubbles.

Two possible disadvantages of the slit catheter are apparent from our studies to date. First, all open-ended catheters without wick fibers are susceptible to the presence of a small air bubble in the catheter's tip just prior to tissue insertion. Such an air bubble seriously reduces catheter response to changes of intracompartmental pressure. However, applying pressure to the syringe after catheter filling and subsequent manipulation of the three-way stopcock (Mubarak et al., 1981) appears to overcome this disadvantage. Second, preliminary studies of tissue fluid sampling indicate that wick catheters are preferable to slit catheters (Hargens, unpublished observations), although this possible disadvantage of the latter does not apply to measurements of intracompartmental pressure in compartment syndromes.

Since most information regarding pressure-time thresholds that necessitate fasciotomy of compartment syndromes is based on measurements of equilibrium tissue fluid pressure by the wick or slit catheter technique, detailed procedures for only these two techniques are given below.

Wick Catheter Procedure

Currently, the best clinical wick catheter system (Fig. 7–6A) combines Dacron suture material and an accurate, reproducible pressure-recording system (Biomedics, Inc.)*. A detailed procedure for setting up this combined system is as follows:

1. Warm up the recorder and transducer for at least 15 minutes to prevent calibration drift.

---

*Wick Catheter™, Biomedics, Inc., 6575 Trinity Court, Dublin, CA 94566.

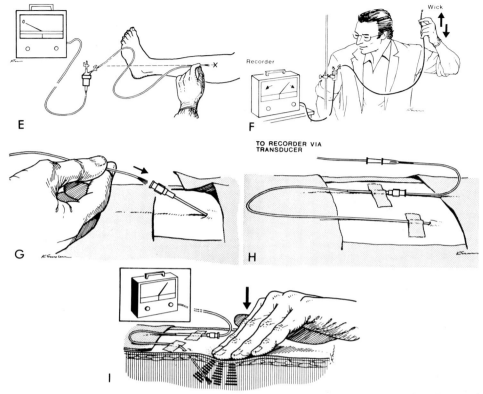

Figure 7–6 *Continued*   *E*, Place tip of wick catheter level with site (*x*) to be measured and have assistant zero system. *F*, Raise the wick catheter tip above insertion site. Pressure should rise and stabilize. If response is sluggish, suspect air bubbles in the line. If pressure falls, suspect leak in system. Lower tip of wick catheter to insertion site level and re-check this zero pressure level. *G*, Insert wick into tissue via plastic sheath, maintaining sterile conditions. *H*, Withdraw plastic sheath and tape catheter to skin. Immediate tissue pressure readings will be obtained. *I*, Check wick catheter response: Palpation over site will cause brisk pressure rise and fall and return to baseline upon relaxation. No infusion of saline is necessary to obtain continuous recordings of intramuscular pressure.

2. While these are warming, prepare the sterile field:
   a. Load lidocaine into a 5-ml syringe.
   b. Load sterile saline solution (20 to 25 ml) into a 30-ml syringe.
   c. Tightly screw the disposable dome onto the transducer. Attach a three-way stopcock tightly to each of the outlets of the dome. Insert saline syringe into one of the stopcocks (Fig. 7–6B).
   d. The stopcock with the syringe attached should be closed to air. Have the second stopcock open to air. Flush the saline solution in through the transducer dome until all the bubbles are cleared through the open stopcock. Close the stopcock off to the syringe and close the second stopcock off to the transducer.
3. Calibration:
   a. Open the stopcock to normal air pressure, set the zero adjust for a zero reading, and watch that the needle does not drift. If it does, the machine is not properly warmed up (Fig. 7–6B).
   b. Once a month check the calibration by connecting a mercury manometer to the stopcock. Turn the stopcock to the manometer and raise the

mercury column to 50 mm Hg. Adjust the gain so that the meter reads 50 mm Hg. If it does not, the meter is not properly warmed up or an air bubble is present in the transducer dome. Check that recorded pressure remains stable at 50 mm Hg. If pressure falls, check for saline leakage. The recorder should now be calibrated.

4. Connect the female end of the manometer tubing to the male end of the stopcock with the 30-ml syringe and fill the tubing, purging all air bubbles (Fig. 7–6B).

5. a. Prep the skin over the desired area with Betadine solution, using sterile technique.

    b. Inject lidocaine into the epidermis and dermis, and within the fascia.

    c. Insert the Jelco catheter placement unit through the skin and fascia at a 45 degree angle; retract the inner steel trocar slightly so that it is fully within the plastic outer catheter. Then, advance the placement unit to the desired intramuscular position (Fig. 7–6C).

6. Wick insertion:

    a. Raise a small drop of saline solution at the end of the manometer tubing and connect the wick. Push the syringe plunger *hard* for 2 to 3 seconds to make sure all bubbles are out of the wick catheter (Fig. 7–6D). Check for air bubbles throughout the saline column.

    b. Hold the tip of the wick catheter at the level of the stopcock (zero point), then raise and lower the wick to verify response to pressure. Place the transducer so that this zero point is level with the anticipated location of the wick in the tissue. Check that the transducer and wick are level by holding the top of the wick at the desired location in the tissue. Adjust the transducer level so that a zero reading is obtained (Fig. 7–6E).

    c. Raise the wick catheter tip above the insertion site, about eye level. Pressure should rise to about 30 to 50 mm Hg and stabilize. If response is sluggish, suspect air bubbles in the lines. If pressure falls, suspect a leak in the system. Lower the tip of the wick catheter level to the insertion site and recheck this zero pressure level (Fig. 7–6F).

    d. Fully withdraw the sharp steel trocar of the Jelco placement unit and insert the wick catheter through the entire length of the plastic outer shield (Fig. 7–6G).

    e. Holding the wick in place, gently retract the outer plastic shield entirely from the tissue. Tape the wick catheter to the skin to maintain wick position (Fig. 7–6H).

    f. Check pressure response by applying gentle finger pressure on the skin over the general area of wick placement. Large pressure deflections should appear on the recorder. If deflections are sluggish, check for air bubbles. If sluggish, consider flushing the wick by turning the stopcock off to the transducer and pushing the syringe plunger slightly. Repeat as necessary (Fig. 7–6I).

7. If the wick reading becomes sluggish or unresponsive, or drifts sharply into the negative pressure range, turn the stopcock off to the transducer and press the syringe plunger slightly. If after this is done a few times the response does not return, the wick should be removed, flushed, and reinserted, or alternatively a new wick catheter should be used.

8. Wick removal: Pull the wick catheter back slowly until the tip has cleared the skin. Check to make sure the wick is still in place. If not, use the monofilament safety line to retrieve wick fibers.

9. Compartment insertion points:
   a. In the leg the midportion of the anterior, lateral, and superficial posterior compartments generally is used. The deep posterior compartment is approached medially by directing the Jelco catheter placement unit posterior to the tibia in the lower third of the leg. "Walk" the needle tip off the posteromedial tibial edge and insert it perpendicular to the long axis of the tibia.
   b. In the forearm, the midportion of volar, dorsal, and mobile wad compartments should be checked.
   c. Avoid measuring the pressure in isolated hematomas as pressures elsewhere in the compartment may be lower. Avoid measuring pressures in plaster cast windows, as local window edema may give a falsely high pressure measurement.
   d. In each compartment it is best to obtain multiple measurements in borderline, elevated pressure situations.
   e. Don't hesitate to measure pressures in control compartments (noninvolved areas) in order to check technique and equipment accuracy.

10. Continuous monitoring vs. repeat pressure measurements: We have recorded compartment pressures continuously for up to 24 hours with the wick catheter technique. For this, sterile, heparinized saline is used (20 units/ml). Occasional flushing of the catheter may be necessary after six to eight hours. However, in the vast majority of patients evaluated for compartment syndromes, we have found that repeat or continuous measurements are not necessary once intracompartmental pressures are documented and correlated with the clinical findings. Furthermore, in borderline cases, we have generally found that repeat measurements of all potentially involved compartments are more useful and practical than the continuous monitoring of one compartment.

Slit Catheter Procedure

The clinical slit catheter and pressure recording system (Howmedica, Inc.)* combines accuracy and precision to ±2 mm Hg and uniformly dynamic response to changes of intracompartmental pressure (Rorabeck et al., 1980). Assembly and insertion of the slit catheter are essentially the same as outlined above for the wick catheter. More care, however, is necessary to avoid an air bubble or air pocket near the tip of the slit catheter. This is accomplished by slightly depressing the syringe plunger after filling the catheter with saline.

The pressure recording meter used with the clinical slit catheter incorporates a number of unique features including a digital display, a variable setting control, and a visual, as well as an audio, warning system that operates if intracompartmental pressure rises above a predetermined value.

Pressure Threshold for Fasciotomy

Based on several clinical (Mubarak et al., 1976, 1978B) and animal (Akeson et al., 1981; Hargens et al., 1981) studies, decompressive fasciotomy is recommended when intracompartmental pressures rise above 30 mm Hg and when there are the

---

*Slit Catheter™, Howmedica, Inc., 359 Veterans Blvd., Rutherford, NJ 07070.

clinical findings of a compartment syndrome. Undoubtedly there exists a spectrum of tolerances to elevated intracompartmental pressure among humans, but in considering the potential dangers we believe that the disastrous sequelae of an unrelieved acute compartment syndrome far outweigh the possibility that a patient may tolerate a pressure over 30 mm Hg without fasciotomy.

As discussed in Chapter 4, previous studies by Whitesides et al. (1975B) and Matsen et al. (1980) suggest that fasciotomies be performed in patients with intracompartmental pressures of 50 to 70 and 45 mm Hg, respectively. Using the needle injection technique, Halpern and Nagel (1979) measured pressures through small openings in plaster casts of fracture patients, and found that intracompartmental pressures of 30 to 40 mm Hg were resolved without fasciotomy. Myoneural necrosis at pressure levels above 30 mm Hg after eight hours, however, is significantly high based on pyrophosphate uptake, muscle histology, and studies of nerve function (Akeson et al., 1981). Unfortunately, it is probable that the pressures measured by Halpern and Nagel (1979) are erroneously high, since we have observed experimentally that any tissue pressure determination made near a small window cut in a cast yields a much higher pressure than one made elsewhere in the compartment under study.

In summary, our clinical and animal studies to date support the conclusion that the threshold intracompartmental pressure at which fasciotomy is recommended is 30 mm Hg for an eight-hour pressurization period. Since the time parameter is usually unknown in most cases of acute compartment syndromes, we recommend that any intracompartmental pressure greater than 30 mm Hg, combined with other positive clinical findings, necessitates fasciotomy. However, one must remember that this threshold pressure of 30 mm Hg is a relative indication for decompression that should be tempered by the following patient factors: overall condition; blood pressure and peripheral perfusion; trend of symptoms and signs; trend of intracompartmental pressures; and the cooperation and reliability of the patient.

OTHER LABORATORY CRITERIA

Blood Tests

Levels of plasma creatine phosphokinase (CPK) are often used as an index of skeletal muscle ischemia and necrosis (Siegel et al., 1975; Chiu et al., 1976). Whereas normal CPK values in human plasma range up to 130 IU (Tietz, 1970), acute compartment syndromes raise plasma CPK to levels from 1000 to 5000 IU, and multiple compartment syndromes as seen in the crush syndrome have plasma CPK levels of 20,000 to 100,000 IU or higher. Unfortunately, blood tests usually indicate that necrosis is already present, and therefore their value as diagnostic tools is somewhat questionable. This applies to other blood parameters that are elevated: white blood count, hematocrit, and serum potassium. Elevation of creatine up to 10 mg/dl from a normal level near 1 mg/dl and blood urea nitrogen at levels between 10 and 150 mg/dl indicate renal failure. Other enzymes that are elevated include aldolase, SGOT, and LDH (Mubarak and Owen, 1975) (see Chapter 11).

Urine Tests

Urinalysis frequently detects presence of myoglobinuria (positive benzidine test for occult blood with absence of red cells). In addition, oliguria (urine output below

400 ml/day) sometimes develops in patients with severe or multiple compartment syndromes (see Chapter 11).

Electromyography and Nerve Conduction

Electromyographic and nerve conduction tests have been utilized primarily in the laboratory investigation of compartment syndromes. Clinically, Matsen and associates (1980) have used a small, battery-powered nerve stimulator to differentiate a direct nerve injury from a compartment syndrome. In patients unable to contract a muscle group voluntarily, this is performed by stimulating the motor nerve that innervates the muscles under consideration at a point just proximal to the muscle compartment. Either sterile needles or surface stimulating electrodes may be employed. Response to this stimulation is reduced or absent when the myoneural junction is rendered ischemic in an acute compartment syndrome. Conversely, normal muscle contraction is observed if a primary neurapraxia is present proximal to the site of nerve stimulation. However, if the nerve injury is located between the stimulation site and the neuromuscular junction, the finding is ambiguous and intracompartmental pressure measurements are necessary to differentiate a primary neurapraxia from an acute compartment syndrome. Matsen and colleagues (1980) note that this technique is not helpful if the patient can voluntarily contract the muscles of the involved compartment, or for prospective monitoring of patients at risk of developing a compartment syndrome.

Peripheral Circulation Assessment

In the investigation of a patient with a possible major artery injury and/or a compartment syndrome, noninvasive studies, such as Doppler blood flow and pulse reappearance time, may be extremely helpful. On other occasions, arteriograms may be necessary. With a typical acute compartment syndrome without an associated arterial injury, the arteriogram will demonstrate patent major arteries with extrinsic compression and closure of the smaller arteries and arterioles (Fig. 7–7).

Venograms have been employed by Reneman (1968) in the evaluation of patients with a possible chronic compartment syndrome (see Chapter 14).

Although laboratory techniques such as radioisotope blood flow studies, muscle pO_2, pCO_2, and pH tests, and technetium pyrophosphate scanning are used in the study of model compartment syndromes, they have not yet become practical in the evaluation of acute compartment syndromes in humans (see Chapter 4).

Compartment Volume Assessment

Assessment of compartment swelling following exercise with the use of ultrasound scanning has recently been accomplished by Gershuni et al. (1981) in our laboratory. However, only normal subjects and chronic compartment syndrome patients have been studied thus far.

Computerized tomography (CT scan) may have a place in the diagnosis and evaluation of the swollen extremity, but quantification of compartment swelling is not of practical value (Fig. 7–8).

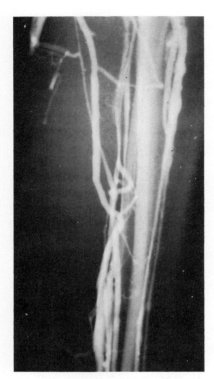

Figure 7–7   Arteriogram: elevated compartmental pressures caused extrinsic compression and closure of the small vessels in this patient's leg.

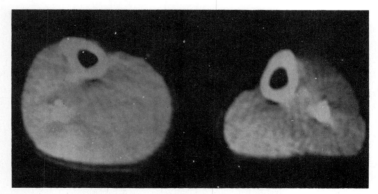

Figure 7–8   Computerized tomography: this may be useful in evaluating a swollen limb. This patient had a superficial and deep posterior compartment syndrome of the left leg.

SUMMARY

The earliest manifestation and sine qua non of a compartment syndrome is elevated intracompartmental pressure. Over a relatively short period of time this increased pressure will cause permanent injury to the myoneural contents of the compartment if left untreated. The treatment of this disorder is relief of the pressure by surgical decompression of the compartment. To achieve early diagnosis and treatment of a compartment syndrome, the best and most direct laboratory test is the measurement of intracompartmental pressure.

REFERENCES

Akeson, W. H., Hargens, A. R., Garfin, S. R., and Mubarak, S. J.: Muscle compartment syndromes and snake bites. *In* Hargens, A. R. (ed.): Tissue Fluid Pressure and Composition. Williams & Wilkins Co., Baltimore, 1981, pp. 215–232.

Brace, R. A., Guyton, A. C., and Taylor, A. E.: A reevaluation of the needle method for measuring interstitial fluid pressure. Am. J. Physiol. 229:603–607, 1975.

Burch, G. E., and Sodeman, W. A.: The estimation of the subcutaneous tissue pressure by a direct method. J. Clin. Invest. 16:845–850, 1937.

Chiu, D., Wang, H. H., and Blumenthal, M. R.: Creatine phosphokinase release as a measure of tourniquet effect on skeletal muscle. Arch. Surg. 111:71, 1976.

Fadnes, H. O., and Aukland, K.: Protein concentration and colloid osmotic pressure of interstitial fluid collected by the wick technique. Microvasc. Res. 14:11–25, 1977.

French, E. B., and Price, W. H.: Anterior tibial pain. Br. Med. J. 2:1291–1296, 1962.

Gershuni, D., Gosink, B. B., Hargens, A. R., Gould, R. N., Forsythe, J. R., Mubarak, S. J., and Akeson, W. H.: Ultrasound scanning to evaluate the anterior musculo-fascial compartment of the leg. Proc. Orthop. Res. Soc., Las Vegas, NV, Feb., 1981.

Guyton, A. C.: A concept of negative interstitial pressure based on pressures in implanted perforated capsules. Circ. Res. 12:399–414, 1963.

Guyton, A. C., Granger, H. J., and Taylor, A. E.: Interstitial fluid pressure. Physiol. Rev. 51:527–563, 1971.

Halpern, A. A., and Nagel, D. A.: Compartment syndromes of the forearm: early recognition using tissue pressure measurements. J. Hand Surg. 4:258–263, 1979.

Hargens, A. R.: Tissue Fluid Pressure and Composition. Williams & Wilkins Co., Baltimore, 1981, 275 pp.

Hargens, A. R., Akeson, W. H., Mubarak, S. J., Owen, C. A., Evans, K. L., Garetto, L. P., Gonsalves, M. R., and Schmidt, D. A.: Fluid balance within the canine anterolateral compartment and its relationship to compartment syndromes. J. Bone Joint Surg. 60–A/:499–505, 1978.

Hargens, A. R., Akeson, W. H., Mubarak, S. J., Owen, C. A., and Garetto, L. P.: Tissue fluid states in compartment syndromes. *In* Lewis, D. H. (ed.): Recent Advances in Basic Microcirculatory Research, Part I. S. Karger, Basel, Bibliotheca Anatomica 15:108–111, 1977A.

Hargens, A. R., Millard, R. W., and Johansen, K.: High capillary permeability in fishes. Comp. Biochem. Physiol. 48–A:675–680, 1974.

Hargens, A. R., Mubarak, S. J., Owen, C. A., Garetto, L. P., and Akeson, W. H.: Interstitial fluid pressure in muscle and compartment syndromes in man. Microvasc. Res. 14:1–10, 1977B.

Hargens, A. R., Romine, J. S., Sipe, J. C., Evans, K. L., Mubarak, S. J., and Akeson, W. H.: Peripheral nerve-conduction block by high muscle-compartment pressure. J. Bone Joint Surg. 61-A:192–200, 1979.

Hargens, A. R., Schmidt, D. A., Evans, K. L., Gonsalves, M. R., Garfin, S. R., Mubarak, S. J., Hagan, P. L., and Akeson, W. H.: Quantitation of skeletal-muscle necrosis in a model compartment syndrome. J. Bone Joint Surg., in press, 1981.

Landerer, A. S.: Die Gewebspannung in ihrem Einfluss auf die örtliche Blutbewegung und Lymphbewegung. Vogel, Leipzig, 1884.

Matsen, F. A., III, Mayo, K. A., Sheridan, G. W., and Krugmire, R. B., Jr.: Monitoring of intramuscular pressure. Surgery 79:702–709, 1976.

Matsen, F. A., III, Winquist, R. A., and Krugmire, R. B.: Diagnosis and management of compartment syndromes in man. J. Bone Joint Surg. 62-A:286–291, 1980.

Matsen, F. A., III, Wyss, C. R., and King, R. V.: The continuous infusion technique in the assessment of clinical compartment syndromes. *In* Hargens, A. R. (ed.): Tissue Fluid Pressure and Composition. Williams & Wilkins Co., Baltimore, 1981, pp. 255–259.

McMaster, P.D.: The pressure and interstitial resistance prevailing in the normal and edematous skin of animals and man. J. Exp. Med. 84:473–494, 1946.

Mubarak, S. J., Hargens, A. R., Lee, Y. F., Lundblad, A-K., Castle, G. S. P., and Rorabeck, C. H.: Slit catheter — a new technique for measuring tissue fluid pressure and quantifying muscle contraction. 27th Annual Meeting, Orthopaedic Res. Soc., Las Vegas, NV, 1981.

Mubarak, S. J., Hargens, A. R., Owen, C. A., and Akeson, W. H.: Muscle pressure measurement with the wick catheter. *In* Goldsmith, H. S. (ed.): Practice of Surgery. Harper & Row, Hagerstown, MD, 1978A, Chap. 20N, pp. 1–8.

Mubarak, S. J., Hargens, A. R., Owen, C. A., Akeson, W. H., and Garetto, L. P.: The wick technique for measurement of intramuscular pressure: a new research and clinical tool. J. Bone Joint Surg. 58-A:1016–1020, 1976.

Mubarak, S. J., and Owen, C. A.: Compartment syndrome and its relation to the crush syndrome: a spectrum of disease. Clin. Orthop. 113:81–89, 1975.

Mubarak, S. J., Owen, C. A., Hargens, A. R., Garetto, L. P., and Akeson, W. H.: Acute compartment syndromes: diagnosis and treatment with the aid of the wick catheter. J. Bone Joint Surg. 60-A:1091–1095, 1978B.

Noddeland, H., Fadnes, H. O., and Aukland, K.: Interstitial protein washdown: an early sign of cardiac failure? Clin. Physiol., submitted, 1981.

Peters, R. M., Hargens, A. R., Utley, J. R., Virgilio, R. W., Rosenkranz, E. R., Zarins, C. K., Menninger, F. J., and Cologne, J. B.: Starling forces following trauma. *In* Hargens, A. R. (ed.): Tissue Fluid Pressure and Composition. Williams & Wilkins Co., Baltimore, 1981, pp. 227–237.

Reneman, R. S.: The Anterior and the Lateral Compartment Syndrome of the Leg. Mouton, The Hague, 1968.

Rorabeck, C. H., Castle, G. S. P., Hardie, R., and Logan, J.: The slit catheter: a new device for measuring intracompartment pressure. Proc. Can. Orthop. Res. Soc., 14th Ann. Meeting, Calgary, Canada, June, 1980, p. 12, and Surgical Forum 31:513, 1980.

Scholander, P. F., Hargens, A. R., and Miller, S. L.: Negative pressure in the interstitial fluid of animals. Science 161:321–328, 1968.

Siegel, B. A., Engel, W. K., and Derrer, E. C.: ^{99m}Tc-diphosphonate uptake in skeletal muscle: a quantitative index of acute damage. Neurology 25:1055–1058, 1975.

Stromberg, D. D., and Wiederhielm, C. A.: Effects of oncotic gradients and enzymes on negative pressures in implanted capsules. Am. J. Physiol. 219:928–932, 1970

Tietz, N. W.: Fundamentals of Clinical Chemistry. W. B. Saunders Co., Philadelphia, 1970, p. 464.

Wells, H. S., Youmans, J. B., and Miller, D. G., Jr.: Tissue pressure (intracutaneous, subcutaneous, and intramuscular) as related to venous pressure, capillary filtration and other factors. J. Clin. Invest. 17:489–499, 1938.

Whitesides, T. E., Jr., Haney, T. C., Hirada, H., Holmes, H. E., and Morimoto, K.: A simple method for tissue pressure determination. Arch. Surg. 110:1311–1313, 1975A.

Whitesides, T. E., Jr., Haney, T. C., Morimoto, K., and Hirada, H.: Tissue pressure measurements as a determinant for the need of fasciotomy. Clin. Orthop. 113:43–51, 1975B.

Wiederhielm, C. A.: Dynamics of transcapillary fluid exchange. J. Gen. Physiol. 52:29–63, 1968.

Wiederhielm, C. A.: The interstitial space and lymphatic pressure in the bat wing. *In* Fishman, A. P., and Hecht, H. H. (eds.): The Pulmonary Circulation and Interstitial Space. University of Chicago Press, Chicago, 1969, pp. 29–41.

Wieherhielm, C. A.: The tissue pressure controversy — a semantic dilemma. *In* Hargens, A. R. (ed.): Tissue Fluid Pressure and Composition. Williams & Wilkins Co., Baltimore, 1981, pp. 21–33.

Wiederhielm, C. A., Woodbury, J. W., Kirk, S., and Rushmer, R. F.: Pulsatile pressures in the microcirculation of frog's mesentery. Am. J. Physiol. 207:173–176, 1964.

Zeluff, G. R.: Absorbable versus nonabsorbable wick material in compartment monitoring. Orthopedic Residents Award Paper, Western Orthop. Assoc., Seattle, WA, Oct. 1978.

Chapter Eight

PRINCIPLES OF TREATING COMPARTMENT SYNDROMES

Scott J. Mubarak, M.D.

PRINCIPLES

The primary mechanism of tissue injury and death of the compartment contents is ischemia secondary to elevated pressure. No satisfactory nonoperative means of treating compartment syndromes has been documented. Surgical decompression, which allows the volume of the compartment to increase, is the only means of pressure relief. Each of the surrounding envelopes of the compartment may play a role in limiting compartmental expansion and maintaining elevated pressure. These envelopes will be discussed (Fig. 8–1).

Cast and Circular Dressings

The volume-restricting effect of casts and circular dressings was first incriminated as the cause of compartmental ischemia by Volkmann himself in 1872 and 1881. Later it was realized that compartment syndromes and Volkmann's contracture could develop without a circular dressing or cast (Murphy, 1914).

The purpose of a plaster cast is to maintain a reduction and immobilize an extremity, both by rigid external support and through soft-tissue volume containment. Using a canine model, Garfin et al. (1980A) compared the relationship between compartmental volume and pressure in casted and uncasted extremities. It was observed that 40 per cent less volume was required to elevate intracompartmental pressures to equivalent levels in casted, as opposed to uncasted, dog hind-limb anterolateral compartments (Figs. 8–2 to 8–5). In a group of dogs fitted with dry cast padding, cast univalving and spreading decreased the pressure by 65 per cent. This procedure is probably sufficient to reduce most of the underlying pressure and symptoms created by the cast in the majority of cases. The tedious job of cutting cast padding accounted for a mean reduction of only 10 per cent. Complete removal of

123

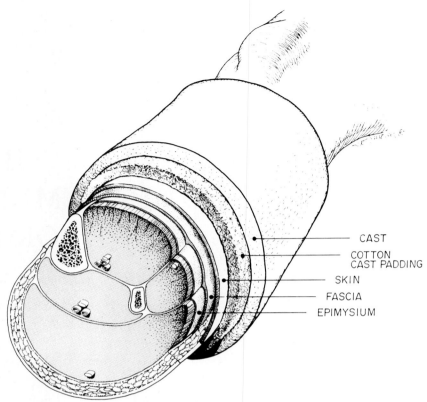

Figure 8–1 The surrounding envelopes of a muscle compartment are illustrated.

CAST
COTTON CAST PADDING
SKIN
FASCIA
EPIMYSIUM

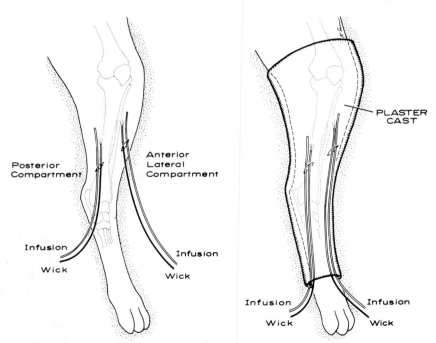

Posterior Compartment

Anterior Lateral Compartment

Infusion

Wick

Infusion

Wick

PLASTER CAST

Infusion

Wick

Infusion

Wick

Figure 8–2 In canine hind limbs, plasma was infused into the anterolateral and posterior compartments while the pressure in these compartments was monitored with the wick catheters. In a large group of these dogs, casts were then applied to determine the degree of volume restriction afforded by the cast. The results are illustrated in Figure 8–3. (From Garfin, S. R., et al.: Quantification of intracompartmental pressure and volume under plaster casts. J. Bone Joint Surg., in press, 1981.)

COMPARTMENTAL PRESSURE AND VOLUME RELATIONSHIPS IN NORMAL LEGS AND WITH LEGS IN CASTS
(mean ± S.E.)

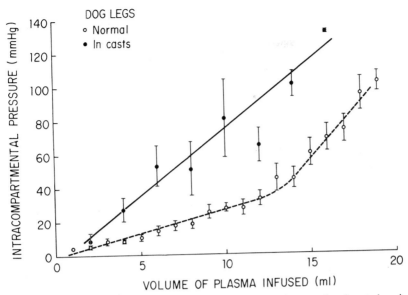

Figure 8-3 Compartmental pressure and volume relationships in normal and casted canine legs. The lower curve illustrates the relationship between volume and pressure in normal, uncasted canine hind-limb anterolateral compartments. The upper curve illustrates the results obtained in casted limbs. Equal volumes caused greater pressure changes in the casted extremities owing to restricted compartment size (approximately 40 per cent). (From Garfin, S. R., et al.: Quantification of intracompartmental pressure and volume under plaster casts. J. Bone Joint Surg., in press, 1981.)

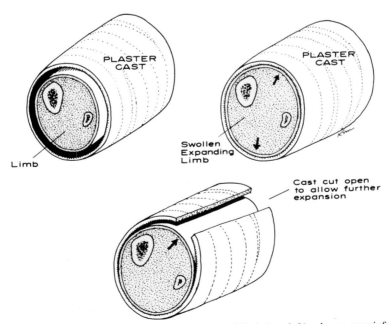

Figure 8-4 After applying the cast to the canine hind limb (*top left*), plasma was infused into the compartments to duplicate the typical pressures found in compartment syndromes (*top right*). While monitoring the pressure, the following procedures were performed (*bottom middle*): (1) cast univalved; (2) cast spread; (3) cast padding cut; and (4) cast removed. The results are illustrated in Figure 8–5. (From Garfin, S. R., et al.: Quantification of intracompartmental pressure and volume under plaster casts. J. Bone Joint Surg., in press, 1981.)

125

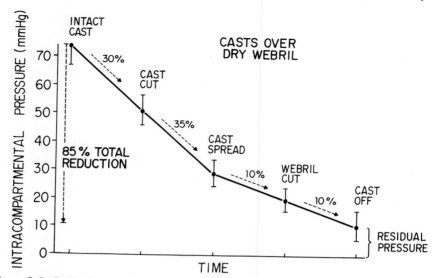

Figure 8–5 Reduction in intracompartmental pressure of casted canine legs with various manipulations, as illustrated: (1) cast univalved — 30 per cent, (2) cast spread — 35 per cent; (3) cast padding cut — 10 per cent, and (4) cast removed — 10 per cent. (From Garfin, S. R., et al.: Quantification of intracompartmental pressure and volume under plaster casts. J. Bone Joint Surg., in press, 1981.)

the cast decreased the pressure to 85 per cent of its previous maximal level. This study demonstrates the effect of the cast on volume containment and pressure elevation, and the necessity of early cast removal in compromised limbs.

Clinically, we have demonstrated similar effects of cast splitting in patients after high tibial osteotomies. Cast splitting and spreading lowered muscle pressure markedly and immediately relieved the symptoms (Fig. 8–6).

Skin

Under some circumstances the skin may be a limiting envelope. Patman and Thompson (1970), although they generally preferred to use multiple small skin incisions for decompression of the leg, recommended extended incisions when

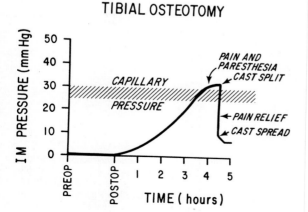

Figure 8–6 Rising anterior compartmental pressure in a patient following high tibial osteotomy. Cast splitting causes a marked fall in the pressure, and relief of symptoms. (From Mubarak, S. J., et al.: The wick catheter technique for measurement of intramuscular pressure. J. Bone Joint Surg., 58-A:1019, 1976.)

massive swelling was present or when there was a delay in therapy. Gaspard et al. (1972) made a distinction between "open fasciotomy, where the skin incision was made to facilitate and ensure complete fascial division, and decompressive dermotomy," which is done after complete fasciotomy, to decompress the limb further. Gaspard et al. did not advocate open fasciotomy in all cases, but rather proposed prompt decompressive dermotomy of the leg, utilizing three longitudinal incisions, if closed fasciotomy had not achieved decompression. In still another report on acute compartment syndromes, Sheridan and Matsen (1976) could demonstrate no significant difference in the complication rate or functional residual with either the open or closed fasciotomy techniques.

Based on our own experience with compartment syndromes, we prefer the limited skin incision in the leg (15 cm) while a more extended incision is employed in the forearm. When monitoring the decompression of the leg intraoperatively, we have noted an 18 per cent mean reduction in pressure from the skin incision alone. This may be compared to a mean decrease of 73 per cent from the fasciotomy of each compartment of the leg (Fig. 8–7). A more extensive dermotomy (see Chapter 10) of 20 cm was necessary on two occasions. In both cases, massive swelling and delay in therapy had occurred.

Fasciotomy

Murphy (1914) was the first to recognize that hemorrhage or edema in muscle within the envelope of fascia could produce pressure ischemia. Using Murphy's suggestion, Jepson (1926) demonstrated in a series of canine experiments that early fasciotomy of the limb would prevent the sequelae of paralysis and contracture. Clinically, Bardenheuer (1911) first documented the value of fasciotomy in the forearm, and later Sirbu et al. (1944) noted its value in the leg. Since 1944, fasciotomy has remained the keystone to decompression of compartment syndromes (Mubarak et al., 1978).

Pressure level and time are two most important variables affecting the functional outcome of the limb. Much experimental work has been performed to investigate these two parameters, and this has been reviewed previously (see Chapter 4). We are interested in determining not only what threshold level of pressure and time causes muscle and nerve injury, but also at what point these changes become irreversible.

Clinically, Sheridan and Matsen (1976) found that fasciotomy performed less than 12 hours after the onset of the compartment syndrome resulted in normal function for 68 per cent of the extremities, compared to only 8 per cent in cases decompressed after 12 hours. Using a canine model, Rorabeck and Clark (1978) demonstrated that fasciotomy restores compartmental blood flow to normal regardless of the time factors, and that, if performed in less than eight hours, nerve conduction velocity also returns to normal at any pressure less than 120 mm Hg.

However, the time element is difficult to evaluate clinically. Unless one has monitored the pressure continuously from the moment of injury, the time at which the pressure becomes elevated to pathologic levels is not known (Fig. 8–8). In our experience, the time between injury and the onset of symptoms (pain and neurologic deficit) of a compartment syndrome may vary from four hours to four days (lag phase). Thus, the time factor is frequently so poorly delineated that the surgeon must correlate only clinical findings and intracompartmental pressure to come to a diagnostic verdict.

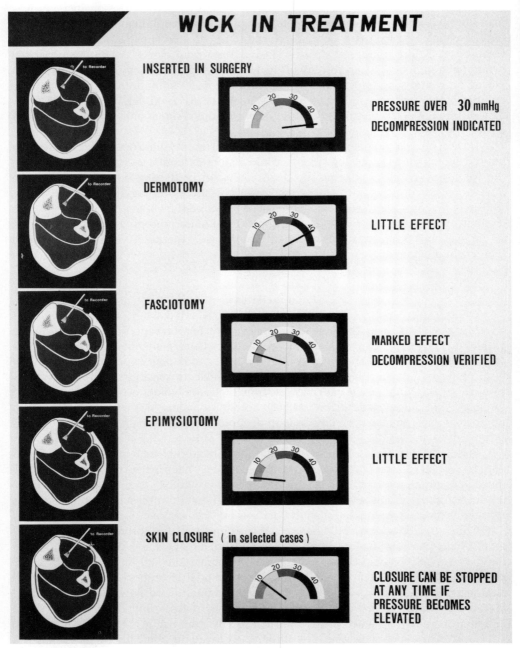

Figure 8–7 Intraoperative use of the wick catheter in patients undergoing decompression demonstrates the effects of dermotomy, fasciotomy, and epimysiotomy. Fasciotomy consistently restored pressures to normal levels. Epimysiotomy was performed in order to demonstrate its value in the decompression. It had a negligible effect except for the gluteus maximus and deltoid muscle compartments. (From Mubarak, S. J., et al.: Acute compartment syndromes: diagnosis and treatment with the aid of the wick catheter. J. Bone Joint Surg. 60-A: 1094, 1978.)

Another question that remains unanswered concerns the possible side effects of a fasciotomy. Does the fascia serve a purpose in maintaining muscle strength? In the canine model we have noted a 20 per cent decrease in acute strength following fasciotomy (Garfin et al., 1980B). We are in the process of studying this finding on a long-term basis to ascertain whether there is improvement in strength with time. If this decline in muscle strength persists, this finding may influence recommendations for fasciotomy in patients with exertional chronic compartment syndromes. Obviously, in the acute compartment syndrome, the benefits of relieving the ischemia by fasciotomy far outweigh the theoretic disadvantage of decreased strength.

Epimysium

Eaton and Green (1972) and Sheridan and Matsen (1976) have noted that the epimysium may be a significant containing envelope. However, none of these authors substantiated their clinical impressions with tissue pressure measurement. Our intraoperative pressure studies have documented only a 2- to 3-mm Hg decrease from the release of this thin muscle covering in the forearm and leg. However, epimysiotomy is necessary to decompress the gluteus maximus or deltoid compartments (Mubarak et al., 1978). In these cases, the fascia is relatively thin and blends with the epimysium, sending septa to form numerous subdivisions within these large multipennate muscles. Thus, multiple fascial-epimysial incisions are necessary to decompress these muscles adequately.

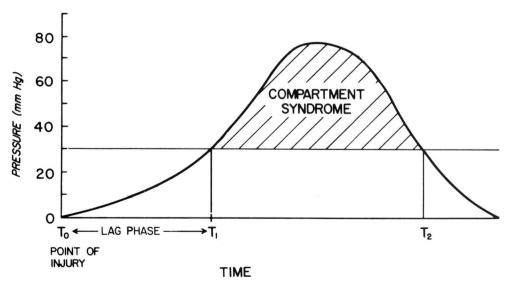

Figure 8-8   The time between injury and the onset of a compartment syndrome may vary from hours to days (lag phase T_0-T_1). The ischemia of the muscle and nerves of the compartment does not take place until the pressure rises to greater than 30 mm Hg (*horizontal line*). Thus, the time from injury to diagnosis and treatment is only a relative indicator of the ischemia period unless one has monitored the tissue pressure from the point of injury. (From Gelberman, R. H., et al.: Compartment syndromes of the forearm: diagnosis and treatment. Clin. Orthop, in press, 1981.

TREATMENT PLAN

Early

When evaluating a patient with a traumatized limb, the physician should carefully document the time of injury and time of both initial and subsequent examinations (Fig. 8–9). These should involve a careful evaluation of circulation, including capillary fill and peripheral pulses. If the swelling does not permit palpation of the pulses, Doppler instrumentation should be used to confirm their presence. Furthermore, an accurate assessment of the peripheral nerve viability of the involved limb should be carried out. The sensory examination should include pinprick and two-point discrimination. These parameters should be monitored frequently by the nursing personnel and treating physician.

In two series of experiments on rabbits, Matsen et al. (1975) have demonstrated that cooling had no effect on postfracture swelling, but that externally applied pressure (maximum 10 mm Hg) by means of air splint tended to reduce swelling (Matsen and Krugmire, 1974). In neither report did these authors advocate altering the approach to humans. In a third series of experiments on humans, however, Matsen et al. (1977) showed that elevation of the legs to 52 cm significantly compromised the anterior tibial arterial pressure at the ankle, and that limb elevation was therefore contraindicated. Similar effects of pressure and elevation on blood flow were noted earlier by Nicholson et al. (1955) and Ashton (1975). We concur with

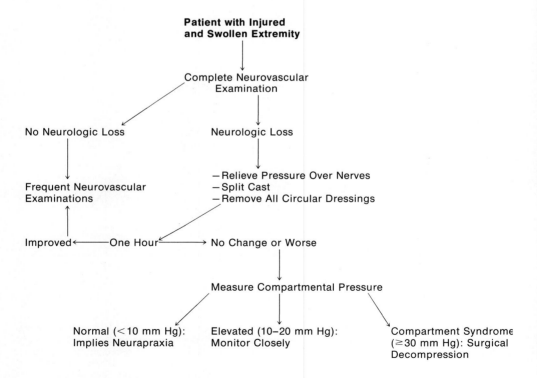

Figure 8–9 Treatment plan of a patient with an injured and swollen extremity.

these findings and recommend that the injured limb be elevated only slightly higher than the patient's heart, to promote venous and lymphatic drainage.

Impending

When a neurologic deficit is observed along with a painfully traumatized limb, one must evaluate and treat the patient promptly. Once again, an accurate assessment of the neurocirculatory status must be obtained. Initially, cast splitting and "windowing" over any involved nerves (i.e., common peroneal) should be performed. If the neurologic deficit persists without improvement for over an hour, removal of the cast and all circular dressings is mandatory.

The next step in the work-up is measurement of intracompartmental pressure. Of the tests available, we feel that this one is best for establishing the diagnosis of a compartment syndrome. Nerve conduction and electromyography may be supportive, but these may simply indicate the state of nerve function and fail to establish etiology. The results of nerve conduction may be particularly confusing if neurapraxia from direct contusion or localized pressure and compartment syndrome coexist. Pressures of less than 30 mm Hg with a nerve deficit suggest an etiology other than compartment syndrome for the neurapraxia (Mubarak et al., 1978).

Acute Compartment Syndrome

Our indications for decompression are:

1. Clinical findings of a compartment syndrome (Chapter 6); and

2. Intracompartmental pressure $\geq$ 30 mm Hg in a normotensive individual (Chapter 7).

As previously noted (Chapter 6), a sensory deficit is the most reliable physical finding. However, the most objective means of diagnosing a compartment syndrome is by a measurement of tissue pressure. Pressure measurement with the wick catheter has been exceedingly helpful in uncooperative, unreliable, or unresponsive patients, and in those with nerve deficit. The wick technique has allowed us to confirm the diagnosis of a compartment syndrome at a very early stage. When clinical and pressure parameters confirm such a diagnosis, immediate surgical intervention should be undertaken. The techniques in the upper and lower extremities are covered subsequently (Chapters 9 and 10).

REFERENCES

Ashton, H.: The effect of increased tissue pressure on blood flow. Clin. Orthop. 113:15–26, 1975.
Bardenheuer, L.: Die Entstehung und Behandlung der ischämischen Muskelkontraktur und Gangrän. Dtsch. Z. Chir. 108:44–201, 1911.
Eaton, R. G., and Green, W. F.: Epimysiotomy and fasciotomy in the treatment of Volkmann's ischemic contracture. Orthop. Clin. North Am. 3:175–185, 1972.
Garfin, S. R., Mubarak, S. J., Evans, K. L., Hargens, A. R., and Akeson, W. H.: Quantification of intracompartmental pressure and volume under plaster casts. Orthop. Trans. 3:17, 1979, and J. Bone Joint Surg., in press, 1981.
Garfin, S. R., Tipton, C. M., Mubarak, S. J., Woo, S. L.-Y., and Hargens, A. R.: The role of fascia in the maintenance of muscle tension and pressure. Trans. Orthop. Res. 4:13, 1979 and J. Appl. Physiol., in press, 1981.

Gaspard, D. J., Cohen, J. L., and Gaspar, M. R.: Decompression dermotomy. A limb salvage adjunct. J. A. M. A. 220:831–833, 1972.

Jepson, P. N.: Ischemic contracture. Experimental study. Am. Surg. 84:785–795, 1926.

Matsen, F. A., and Krugmire, R. B.: The effect of externally applied pressure on post fracture swelling. J. Bone Joint Surg. 56-A:1586–1591, 1974.

Matsen, F. A., Mayo, K. A., Krugmire, R. B., Sheridan, G. W., and Kraft, G. H.: A model compartmental syndrome in man with particular reference to the quantification of nerve function. J. Bone Joint Surg. 59-A:648–653, 1977.

Matsen, F. A., Questad, K., and Matsen, A. L.: The effect of local cooling on post fracture swelling. A controlled study. Clin. Orthop. 109:201–206, 1975.

Mubarak, S. J., Hargens, A. R., Owen, C. A., Garetto, L. P., and Akeson, W. H.: The wick catheter technique for measurement of intramuscular pressure: a new research and clinical tool. J. Bone Joint Surg. 58-A:1016, 1020, 1976.

Mubarak, S. J., Owen, C. A., Hargens, A. R., Garetto, L. P., and Akeson, W. H.: Acute compartment syndromes: diagnosis and treatment with the aid of the wick catheter. J. Bone Joint Surg. 60-A:1091–1095, 1978.

Murphy, J. B.: Myositis. J. A. M. A. 63:1249–1255, 1914.

Nicholson, J. T., Foster, R. M., and Heath, R. D.: Bryant's traction: a provocative cause of circulatory complications. J. A. M. A. 157:415–418, 1955.

Patman, R. D., and Thompson, J. E.: Fasciotomy in peripheral vascular surgery. Arch. Surg. 101:663–670, 1970.

Rorabeck, C. H., and Clark, K. M.: The pathophysiology of the anterior tibial compartment syndrome: an experimental investigation. J. Trauma 18:229–304, 1978.

Sheridan, G. W., and Matsen, F. A.: Fasciotomy in the treatment of the acute compartment syndrome. J. Bone Joint Surg. 58-A:112–115, 1976.

Sirbu, A. B., Murphy, M. J., and White, A. S.: Soft tissue complications of fractures of the leg. Calif. West. Med. 60:53–56, 1944.

Volkmann, R. von: Krankenheiten der Bewegungsorgane. *In* Handbuch der Chirurgie, Pitha-Billroth 2:846, 1872.

Volkmann, R. von: Die ischaemischen Muskellähmungen und Kontrakturen. Zentralb. Chir. 8:801, 1881.

Chapter Nine

UPPER EXTREMITY COMPARTMENT SYNDROMES: TREATMENT

Richard H. Gelberman, M.D.

INTRODUCTION

Decompression of a forearm compartment syndrome was first recommended many years after the serious effects of established Volkmann's contracture had been appreciated. Bardenheuer (1911) was the first to report on fasciotomy in the forearm. This procedure, originally called aponeurectomy, consisted of a division of the deep fascia of the antecubital fossa and forearm. Other authors (Murphy, 1914; Jorge, 1925; Jepson, 1926; Moulonquet and Seneque, 1928; Massart, 1935) stressed the need for fasciotomy in certain patients, but none of these authors described a specific operative technique. Garber (1939) recommended decompression of forearm compartment syndromes with release of the aponeurotic sheaths of the flexor muscles, along with exploration of the median and ulnar nerves and the brachial artery and its major branches. He did not describe his specific skin and fascial incisions, however.

Benjamin (1957) briefly reported a surgical technique used for several cases of impending Volkmann's ischemic contracture. He recommended a transverse division of the fascia of the antecubital fossa, followed by a longitudinal division of the deep fascia of the forearm. Benjamin also suggested that other areas may need decompression, but he did not indicate which areas or how they might be determined.

Eichler and Lipscomb (1967) described an approach to the patient with impending Volkmann's contracture in greater detail. They outlined a stepwise scheme that included a division of forearm skin, subcutaneous tissue, and fascia. Eaton and Green (1972) concentrated in more detail on the forearm anatomy, and described a specific operative technique. Their skin incision began distal to the elbow flexion crease, medial to the biceps tendon, and was extended distally in the longitudinal axis of the midforearm, to the transverse flexion crease at the wrist. The antebrachial fascia was incised longitudinally along its full length. The epimysium of all poorly vascularized muscles was then sectioned in a distal-to-proximal direction. Compromised muscles were explored and decompressed. The fascia was left open, and delayed closure with split-thickness skin grafts and relaxing incisions was performed 48 to 72 hours later.

Neumeyer and Kilgore (1976) reported their experience with 14 patients who had forearm compartment syndromes. Although these authors did not discuss their technique, they described their incision pictorially. It began adjacent to the medial epicondyle, extended obliquely across the antecubital fossa over the volar mobile wad,* and returned to the midline in the distal forearm. It continued in a curvilinear fashion across the carpal canal to the midpalm. This report recommends wide exposure of all three possible areas of involvement — the flexor or extensor compartments of the forearm and the intrinsics of the hand. Closure was accomplished by split skin grafting after several days.

Whitesides and associates (1975) described another operative approach. Their incision began above the elbow laterally, and was carried transversely across the antecubital fossa to the proximal-medial forearm. It was continued distally along the ulnar border of the forearm to the wrist, where it curved laterally in the flexor crease of the wrist, and extended into the palm in the thenar crease. The fascia was opened from above the elbow to the midpalm. The carpal tunnel and all neurovascular and muscular envelopes were opened fully. The advantage of the volar-ulnar approach is that the flexor tendons and median nerve are not left exposed in the distal forearm. Whitesides warned that a subcutaneous fasciotomy should never be performed in the forearm. The fascia is left open, and closed by split-thickness skin grafting 48 to 72 hours later.

Since 1976 we have employed a single, longitudinal, curvilinear incision for decompression of the volar forearm. It is designed for division of the volar antebrachial fascia and transverse carpal ligament, as well as exposure of the arteries and nerves of the forearm and the mobile wad. The incision is nearly identical to McConnell's combined exposure of the median and ulnar neurovascular bundles, as described by Henry (1973).

VOLAR AND DORSAL FASCIOTOMY OF FOREARM

Background

Initially we evaluated the effectiveness of the volar forearm fasciotomy in a series of cadaver experiments (Gelberman et al., 1978). Plasma was infused into the volar, dorsal, and mobile wad regions of 15 fresh cadaver limbs. The pressure in the three regions was monitored by the wick catheter technique, while a variety of volar and dorsal incisions were used to carry out fasciotomies. The major volar incisions made were the volar-ulnar incision described by Whitesides et al. (1975) and the curvilinear, midline volar incision (Fig. 9–1). Both were effective in lowering pressures in the volar forearm, and both also lowered pressures within the mobile wad and dorsal regions in approximately one half of the limbs. The volar forearm pressure generally fell to normal values when the antebrachial fascia had been

---

*Mobile wad (of Henry)—term used to describe brachioradialis and extensor carpi radialis longus and brevis muscles.

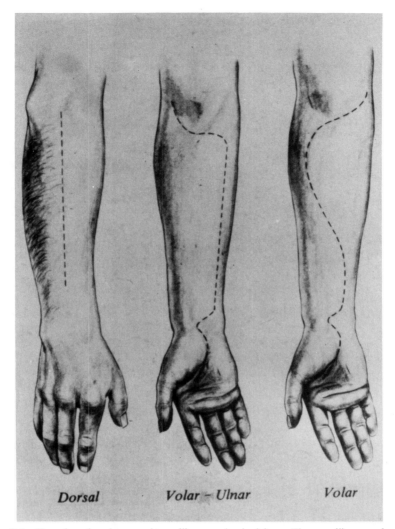

Figure 9–1 Dorsal, volar-ulnar, and curvilinear volar incisions. The curvilinear volar incision is preferred because of the exposure afforded to major nerves, brachial artery, and mobile wad. (With permission from Gelberman, R. H., et al.: Decompression of forearm compartment syndromes. Clin. Orthop. 134:225–229, 1978.)

divided from the lacertus fibrosus to the junction of the middle and distal thirds of the forearm. When the dorsal pressures remained elevated following volar fasciotomy, a dorsal fasciotomy was performed (Fig. 9–1). The dorsal fasciotomy was effective in lowering dorsal and mobile wad pressure in the remaining limbs.

Since 1976 the adequacy of forearm decompression has been monitored intraoperatively with the wick catheter in 15 patients.

Instruments

Instruments for this procedure include the scalpel, right-angled retractors, and small Metzenbaum scissors. Fasciotomes are not recommended for use in the forearm because of the subcutaneous location of the major nerves and arteries.

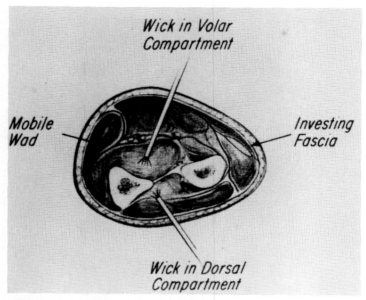

Figure 9–2 Cross-section of the proximal forearm demonstrating placement of wick catheters. (With permission from Gelberman, R. H., et al.: Decompression of forearm compartment syndromes. Clin. Orthop. 134:225–229, 1978.)

Volar Approach

A complete, single skin incision, beginning proximal to the antecubital fossa and extending to the midpalm, can be utilized for volar forearm decompression. It is highly advisable that tissue pressure measurements be available intraoperatively. Volar and dorsal pressures are measured prior to the skin incision (Fig. 9–2). The incision begins 1 cm proximal and 2 cm lateral to the medial epicondyle, and is carried obliquely across the antecubital fossa and over the volar aspect of the mobile wad. It is gently curved medially, reaching the midline at the junction of the middle and distal thirds of the forearm (Fig. 9–3), and is continued straight distally to the proximal wrist crease, just ulnar to the palmaris longus tendon. The forearm incision is extended across the volar wrist crease in the curvilinear fashion. It is carried no further radially than the midaxis of the ring finger, to avoid injury to the palmar cutaneous branch of the median nerve. The incision is terminated in the midpalm at a level even with the base of the thumb-index web. The carpal tunnel has been released in all of our cases, and we now recommend this as a standard part of forearm decompression.

In cases with median nerve dysfunction, in addition to the carpal tunnel release, the median nerve should be explored in the proximal forearm. There are three areas of potential neural compression in the proximal forearm. The most proximal, the lacertus fibrosus, is always released as part of the fasciotomy. The next area of possible compression is the proximal edge of the pronator teres, and the third is the proximal edge of the flexor digitorum superficialis. The surgeon should be certain that the nerve lies free in all three regions.

It is possible to avoid the long, continuous volar incision by dividing it into separate proximal and distal incisions. The proximal incision begins in the same

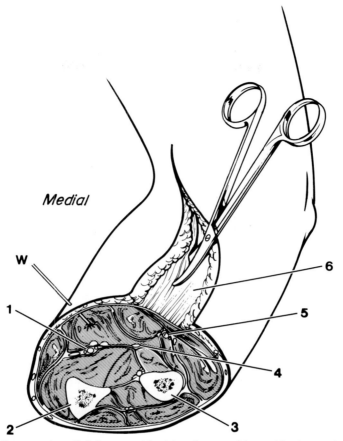

Figure 9–3   Cross-section of left forearm with wick catheter position and fasciotomy incision illustrated. W = wick catheter; 1 = ulnar nerve; 2 = ulna; 3 = radius; 4 = median nerve; 5 = radial artery; 6 = forearm fascia. (With permission from Gelberman, R. H., et al.: Compartment syndromes of the forearm: diagnosis and treatment. Clin. Orthop. in press, 1981.)

manner, but may be terminated in the midforearm where the digital flexors become predominantly tendinous (Fig. 9–4). A standard carpal tunnel incision, beginning just proximal to the proximal wrist crease, is the second incision. This leaves approximately 10 cm in the distal forearm where the fascia is not incised.

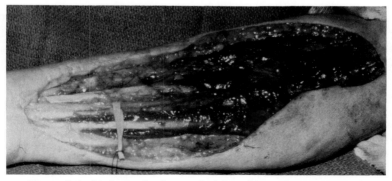

Figure 9–4   Limited volar forearm incision with median nerve tagged.

These two incisions have the advantage of less muscle and tendon exposure, and the skin edges do not retract as much as with the continuous incision. The brachial artery and median nerve can be isolated and decompressed in the elbow region and proximal forearm, and the median nerve can be decompressed at the wrist. Delayed primary closure has not been possible in most instances, however, and split-thickness grafting, although less extensive, has been necessary even with the two incisions.

The chief disadvantage of two incisions is that a complete forearm fasciotomy is not performed. Approximately 10 cm of fascia is left intact in the distal forearm. The intact fascia and skin may prove to be significant, and unless forearm pressures can be monitored during the operative procedure, and a satisfactory reduction of pressures demonstrated, the long, continuous incision is recommended.

Dorsal Approach

Following the volar fasciotomy, the pressure in the dorsal compartment is remeasured. If the pressure exceeds 30 mm Hg, a dorsal fasciotomy is performed. The incision begins 2 cm lateral and 2 cm distal to the lateral epicondyle (Fig. 9–1). It is extended straight distally toward the midline of the wrist for 7 to 10 cm, depending on the size of the forearm. The skin edges are undermined, and the dorsal fascia incised directly in line with the skin incision. Pressures are then determined in the dorsal and mobile wad regions. An additional incision for the mobile wad has not been necessary in any of our cases. Furthermore, the mobile wad area can be exposed easily with the curvilinear volar incision.

This procedure completes the decompression of the volar and dorsal regions of the forearm. If intraoperative pressure monitoring has been performed, a final pressure in each compartment is checked. The wounds are packed open, and a bulky, compressive hand dressing extending above the elbow with plaster forearm and elbow splints is applied. Skin incisions are not closed at the time of fasciotomy.

If the diagnosis was delayed and some muscle appears necrotic, a superficial debridement is carried out. More definitive debridements are carried out secondarily when muscle viability can be determined more accurately.

After Care

The extremity is elevated continuously in the bulky dressing. At three to four days postfasciotomy the patient is returned to the operating room. The skin of the hand and wrist and the proximal few centimeters of the wound can frequently be closed at this time. The large central portion of the wound can be skin-grafted at this time, or can be treated by progressive Steri-Strip closure to decrease the size of the wound. Ultimately, skin grafts have been needed in all of our cases (Figs. 9–5 to 9–7).

If some of the forearm musculature is necrotic, further debridement is carried out every three to four days until the granulating bed is healthy. Quantitative cultures are used to determine the appropriate time for grafting.

Active and active assisted range of motion of the hand is started on the second

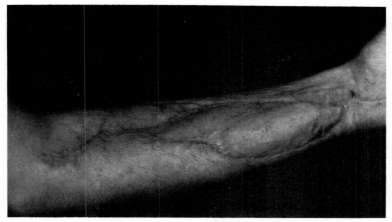

Figure 9–5   Case 1. Volar forearm fasciotomy following partial closure and split-thickness skin grafting.

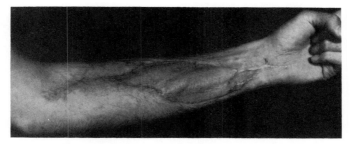

Figure 9–6   Case 1. Digital flexion is illustrated.

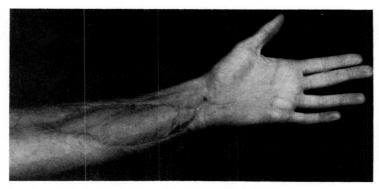

Figure 9–7   Case 1. Digital extension is illustrated.

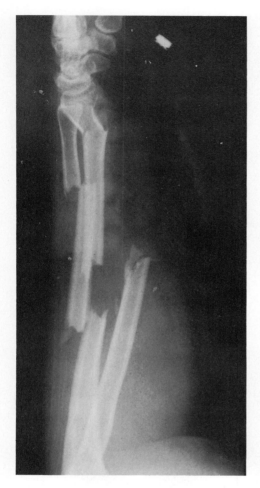

Figure 9–8 Case 2. Segmental fractures of the radius and ulna associated with forearm compartment syndromes. The volar pressure was 80 mm Hg, and the dorsal pressure 35 mm Hg prior to decompression.

day postfasciotomy, while the patient is still in the bulky dressing. Exercises are discontinued for seven days after split skin grafting is performed, and then reinstituted. The bulky dressing is discontinued at two and one half to three weeks, and the patient is placed in a thermoplastic splint with the thumb in opposition and the wrist neutral. The elbow is left free.

FRACTURES OF RADIUS AND ULNA AND
COMPARTMENT SYNDROMES OF FOREARM

Acute forearm compartment syndromes are sometimes associated with fractures of the radius and ulna. In many cases, internal fixation of both bones should be undertaken at the time of fasciotomy (Figs. 9–8 to 9–10). If the fractures are open and contaminated, however, the fasciotomy is performed, and the wound is debrided and irrigated copiously. The fractures are then supported in a bulky dressing with plaster

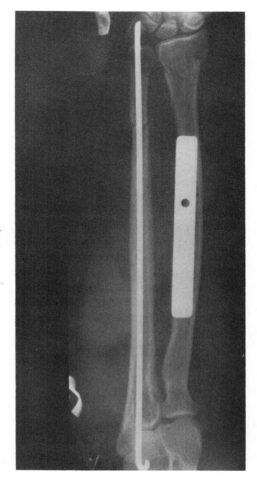

Figure 9–9 Case 2. Internal fixation of the radius and ulna fractures was carried out at the time of forearm decompression. Anteroposterior radiograph.

splints. Skin grafting is carried out when the granulating bed is fresh, as described above. Delayed internal fixation of both bones may be performed two to three weeks later.

Other options are available for managing forearm fractures associated with compartment syndromes. External fixation may prove to be effective in some instances, but we have not used this method. A potential minor disadvantage is difficulty with skin mobilization for partial wound closure. Conservative methods with long arm casts or functional bracing techniques may be advisable in some cases.

PROPHYLACTIC FASCIOTOMY OF FOREARM

There are situations in which prophylactic forearm fasciotomy may be advisable. Forearm compartment syndromes sometimes develop after arterial reconstruc-

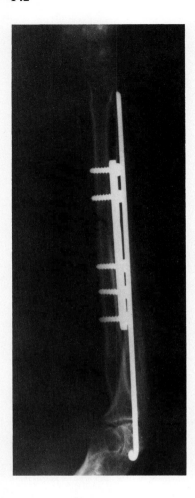

Figure 9–10   Case 2. Lateral radiograph of forearm.

tions, but the forearm fasciotomy should be reserved for circumstances in which the wick catheter reading is abnormally elevated (>30 mm Hg). The patient's condition should be followed closely for any signs of increasing pressure.

This plan is like that for similar situations in the leg in which the double-incision fasciotomy has been recommended prophylactically. Compartment syndromes following arterial reconstruction occur more frequently in the lower extremity, and the leg decompression is a smaller, less extensive operation.

SUPRACONDYLAR FRACTURES AND COMPARTMENT SYNDROMES OF FOREARM

Supracondylar fractures may be associated with forearm compartment syndromes (Fig. 9–11). The fracture should be reduced by closed methods in the operating room. If forearm pressures are elevated following reduction, a fasciotomy is carried out (Fig. 9–12). The fracture then is best treated by percutaneous pin fixation or overhead olecranon pin traction. Wound management is identical to that described earlier for forearm fasciotomy.

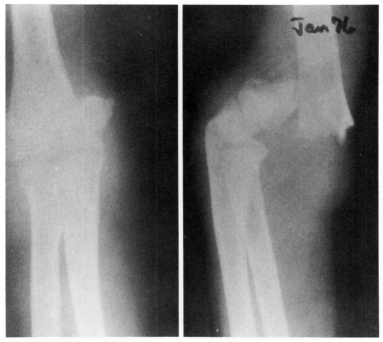

Figure 9–11 Markedly displaced supracondylar fracture associated with a forearm compartment syndrome.

ARTERIAL INJURIES AND COMPARTMENT
SYNDROMES OF FOREARM

Arterial injuries associated with compartment syndromes most often occur following supracondylar fractures, forearm fractures, or external penetrating injuries. These are complex injuries for which the most systematic approach is indicated (Fig. 9–12). If an arterial injury associated with a compartment syndrome and fracture is suspected, the patient should be taken immediately to the operating room. In an adult, axillary block anesthesia is beneficial. In a child, general anesthesia followed by an axillary block is indicated. The regional block performs two important functions. First, it has a vasodilating effect, which is helpful if the collateral circulation is in spasm. Second, if an arterial repair is carried out, it assists by maintaining maximal lumen size in the injured vessel.

The fracture should next be reduced, and the pulses and hand circulation reassessed. Volar and dorsal and, if necessary, hand pressures should then be measured with the wick catheter. If the pressures are elevated, a volar forearm fasciotomy is carried out. The brachial, radial, and ulnar arteries are then explored. Fasciotomy alone will not prevent ischemic injury unless the arterial circulation is fortuitously or deliberately restored by the surgeon.

If the artery is trapped in a fracture site, it is freed and cleansed of any surrounding hematoma. If a segment of the artery is in spasm, it should first be cleansed meticulously. Topical papaverine (2½ per cent) or lidocaine (1 per cent) is often helpful in clearing the spasm. It may take 20 to 30 minutes for the spasm to improve significantly. If a segment of the artery is irreparably damaged or lacerated,

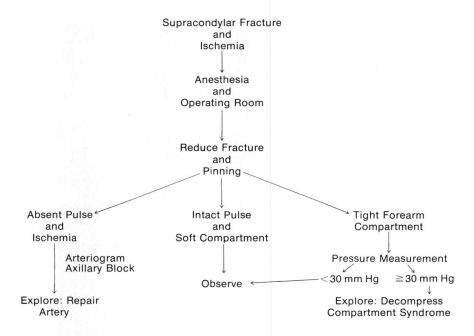

Figure 9–12   Schema for management of supracondylar fractures associated with upper extremity ischemia.

it may be managed in one of two ways. The brachial artery may be excised in the area of injury, and ligated proximally and distally. Collateral circulation about the elbow is generally profuse, and hand circulation most often remains adequate. If either the radial or ulnar artery is lacerated singly, it may also be ligated. If both forearm arteries are lacerated, they must be repaired. Repair of lacerated brachial arteries is also recommended, but whether this is done or not, the surgeon must be certain that hand circulation is adequate before leaving the operating room.

In certain situations in which an arterial injury is suspected, but the location is in doubt, a preoperative transfemoral-brachial arteriogram may be helpful.

COMPARTMENT SYNDROMES OF HAND

Background and Findings

An acute compartment syndrome of the hand leading to an ischemic contracture was first described by Finochietto (1920). A characteristic syndrome associated with the acute compartment syndrome in the hand has subsequently been recognized. The patient generally presents with hand pain following a crush injury, compression syndrome, or forearm vascular injury. Spinner et al. (1972) have described the diagnostic triad of pain, intrinsic paralysis, and increasing pain on stretching the involved intrinsic muscle. The hand has an intrinsic minus attitude, with metacarpophalangeal joint hyperextension and interphalangeal joint flexion. It is grossly edematous and tender. Sensation is generally normal, but if it is diminished carpal tunnel involvement should be suspected. There may be electromyographic evidence of intrinsic muscle denervation as early as nine to ten days postinjury. The process may involve one or all intrinsic compartments, and may be acute or may persist in a subacute form for days or weeks. If untreated, an irreversible muscle necrosis occurs. The hand compartment syndrome may be differentiated from the forearm compartment syndrome, in which pain is increased only on stretching the involved flexor muscles. Passive abduction and adduction of the digits demonstrates intrinsic compression (see Chapter 3).

Treatment

The wick catheter may be used to document an increase in pressure. A pressure greater than 30 mm Hg is an indication for fasciotomy. The most commonly involved compartments of the hand are the interossei. The dorsal decompression is performed through longitudinal incisions in the intermetacarpal spaces (Fig. 9–13). On incision of the dorsal fascia, the interosseous muscles generally bulge out through the wound. The adductor is decompressed by the incision of the dorsal thumb web space. The wounds are left open and the hand is placed in a long-arm, bulky dressing. After 48 to 72 hours of continuous elevation, the patient is returned to the operating room for wound closure.

COMPARTMENT SYNDROMES OF ARM AND SHOULDER

Compartment syndromes above the elbow in the biceps, triceps, and deltoid regions are usually seen in patients following drug overdose-limb compression. Besides the local condition of the compartment syndrome, these patients also frequently demonstrate the systemic problems of the crush syndrome.

The anterior brachium may be decompressed by a longitudinal, anteromedial incision. The posterior brachium is decompressed by a straight posterior, longitudinal incision. With deltoid muscle involvement, the same principles are employed as in

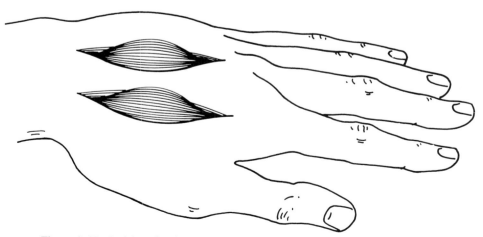

Figure 9–13   Incisions for decompression of compartment syndromes in the hand.

treatment of the gluteus maximus (Chapter 10). The deltoid is a multipennate muscle divided by multiple septa of the combined fascia and epimysium layer. To adequately decompress this muscle compartment, multiple incisions are necessary in the fascia-epimysium (see Figs. 11–12 to 11–17). Again, tissue pressure measurement is extremely valuable in order to document the adequacy of decompression.

REFERENCES

Bardenheuer, L.: Die Entstehung und Behandlung der ischämischen Muskelkontractur und Gangrän. Dtsch. Z. Chir. 108:44, 1911.
Benjamin, A.: The relief of traumatic arterial spasm in threatened Volkmann's ischaemic contracture. J. Bone Joint Surg. 39-B:711, 1957.
Eaton, R. G., and Green, W. T.: Epimysiotomy and fasciotomy in treatment of Volkmann's ischemic contracture. Orthop. Clin. North Am. 3:175, 1972.
Eichler, G. R., and Lipscomb, P. R.: The changing treatment of Volkmann's ischemic contractures from 1955 to 1965 at the Mayo Clinic. Orthop. Clin. North Am. 50:215, 1967.
Finochietto, R.: Volkmann's contracture of the intrinsic muscles of the hand. Bol. y trab. Soc. Cir. (Buenos Aires) 4:31, 1920.
Garber, J. N.: Volkmann's contracture of fractures of the forearm and elbow. J. Bone Joint Surg. 21:154, 1939.
Gelberman, R. H., Zakaib, G. S., Mubarak, S. J., Hargens, A. R., and Akeson, W. H.: Decompression of forearm compartment syndromes. Clin. Orthop. 134:225, 1978.
Henry, A. K.: Extensile Exposure. 2nd ed. Churchill Livingstone, Edinburgh and London, 1973.
Jepson, P. N.: Ischemic contracture. Ann. Surg. 84:785, 1926.
Jorge, J.: Rétraction ischémique de Volkmann. Rapport d'Albert Monchet. Bull. Mem. Soc. Nat. Chir. 51:884, 1925.
Massart, R.: La maladie de Volkmann. Rev. Orthop. 3, Ser. 22:385, 1935.
Moulonquet, P., and Seneque, J.: Syndrome de Volkmann. Bull. Mem. Soc. Nat. Chir. 54:1094, 1928.
Murphy, J. B.: Myositis. J.A.M.A. 63:1249, 1914.
Neumeyer, W. L., and Kilgore, E. S., Jr.: Volkmann's ischemic contracture due to soft tissue injury alone. J. Hand Surg. 1:221, 1976.
Spinner, M., Aiache, A., Silver, L., and Barsky, A.: Impending ischemic contracture of the hand. Plast. Reconstr. Surg. 50:341, 1972.
Whitesides, T. E., Jr., Haney, T. C., Morimoto, K., and Harada, H.: Tissue pressure measurements as a determinant for the need for fasciotomy. Clin. Orthop. 113:43, 1975.

Chapter Ten

LOWER EXTREMITY COMPARTMENT SYNDROMES: TREATMENT

Scott J. Mubarak, M.D.

INTRODUCTION

Sirbu et al. (1944) were among the first to report on fasciotomy of the leg, after successfully treating an acute exertional compartment syndrome. Dennis (1945) utilized two incisions (medial and lateral) of the leg and thigh to decompress compartment syndromes in a patient following vein ligation. DeBakey and Simeone (1946), in an analysis of 2,471 arterial injuries in World War II, briefly discussed their technique of surgical decompression. They described the medial and lateral leg incisions made, but did not go into any detail regarding compartment anatomy.

In 1966, Seddon noted that the deep posterior compartment was frequently involved and inadequately treated. This report initiated the concept of four anatomic compartments of the leg that needed specific surgical decompression. Kelly and Whitesides (1967) stressed the anatomic importance of the four compartments, and suggested that fibulectomy-fasciotomy through a single lateral incision was an adequate means of decompressing these compartments. The specific details of this procedure were outlined more completely by Ernst and Kaufer (1971).

Patman and Thompson (1970) favored fibulectomy for: (1) severe cases; (2) cases with obvious myonecrosis or paralysis; and (3) those in which fibulectomy would aid exposure and repair of a distal popliteal artery. They also advocated the double-incision method through a more limited incision in milder cases, and for prophylaxis against impending compartment syndromes. The importance of decompressing the deep posterior compartment was emphasized. A similar recommendation for two incisions in postischemic compartment syndromes was made by Jacob (1974).

Matsen and Clawson (1975) recommended a skin incision over the lower third of the leg as an approach to the deep posterior compartment. More recently, Matsen and Krugmire (1978) suggested a single lateral incision (parafibular approach) for decompressing all four compartments. This is similar to the technique suggested by Willhoite and Moll (1970).

Since 1974 we have employed the double-incision technique for decompression of the leg (Mubarak and Owen, 1977). This procedure is desiged to gain access via two incisions to any or all of the four compartments of the leg when these are involved with acute or chronic compartment syndromes.

DOUBLE-INCISION FASCIOTOMY OF LEG

Background

We initially compared double-incision fasciotomy to fibulectomy-fasciotomy in a series of cadaver experiments (Mubarak and Owen, 1977). Saline was infused into the four compartments of the cadaveric legs to elevate the pressure. Next, while pressure was continuously monitored in the compartments, either a double-incision fasciotomy or a fibulectomy-fasciotomy was performed. Both techniques, when properly performed, proved equally effective in decompressing the limb. With the fibulectomy technique, the approach to the fibula effectively decompressed the lateral and superficial posterior compartments. Subperiosteal, subtotal fibulectomy decreased the pressure in the anterior and deep posterior compartments by only 10 to 15 mm Hg from preoperative levels. Removal of the fibula was not enough to decompress these two compartments. The pressure fell to normal only when the entire length of the fibular periosteal bed was opened in each compartment, as in the technique described by Ernst and Kaufer (1971). This portion of the procedure was somewhat difficult owing to the distortion of the anatomy after fibulectomy and soft-tissue swelling.

In practice we have used the double-incision fasciotomy on more than 40 patients since 1974. In most of these we have verified the adequacy of decompression and the technique with intraoperative pressure monitoring. The only modifications we have made from our original description have been in regard to the length of the skin incision, and this is discussed below.

We feel that the major advantages of the double-incision technique over fibulectomy-fasciotomy are:

1. It is simpler and requires minimal dissection. The procedure can be performed under local anesthesia if necessary. This is especially important in treating patients who have compartment syndromes resulting from drug overdose-limb compression, or arterial disease with postischemic swelling. These individuals often are extremely ill and are poor anesthetic risks.

2. It is faster and relatively safer. Both procedures require close attention to anatomic detail in order to avoid damaging important cutaneous nerves. However, the double-incision method involves less risk, primarily because the fascial incisions are all superficial and avoid deep neurovascular structures.

3. The fibula is left intact. Concern by surgeons involving the sequelae of fibulectomy in a child or an adult may lead to procrastination, with potentially disastrous results. Fibulectomy-fasciotomy, being a much larger operation, may not be performed in the borderline cases or prophylactically.

The major advantages over fasciotomies performed through long, single skin incisions (Willhoite and Moll, 1970; Matsen and Krugmire, 1978) are:

1. Two more limited skin incisions offer better cosmesis, as delayed primary closure can usually be performed at around one week. In over 90 per cent of our cases, skin grafting has not been required.

2. Any portion of the double-incision technique may be used for decompression of any specific combination of compartments fewer than four.

3. Two incisions provide an opportunity to perform a double decompressive dermotomy if this is required (Gaspard et al., 1972). In these rare cases when the skin is a limiting envelope, a single incision may not be enough for complete decompression, and therefore double decompressive dermotomies will be required.

4. Debridement is facilitated through these skin incisions if necrotic muscle is encountered.

Instruments

Necessary instruments for this procedure include right-angled retractors (army-navy), 12-inch Metzenbaum scissors, and/or a fasciotome (Fig. 10–1). We have developed a commercially available fasciotome* modified from the instruments suggested by others (Mozes et al., 1962; Rosato et al., 1966; Bate, 1972). This instrument is designed to incise the fascia without the need for a skin incision along the whole length of the leg.

Skin Incisions

A limited skin incision approximately 15 cm long (roughly one third the length of the leg) can be utilized for both the anterolateral and posteromedial incisions. This is best if the compartment syndrome is diagnosed and treated promptly. If the limited approach is utilized, it is highly advisable that intraoperative tissue pressure measurement be used to document the adequacy of decompression (Mubarak et al., 1978).

Our limited incision technique has the advantages of less muscle exposure, and the skin edges do not retract as much as with extensive incision. Because of this

---

*Made by Down Surgical Co., Toronto, Ont., Canada.

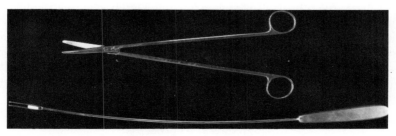

Figure 10–1 A 12-inch Metzenbaum scissors and/or a fasciotome are useful instruments for decompression of the leg, utilizing double-incision fasciotomy technique. (With permission from Mubarak, S. J., and Hargens, A. R.: Diagnosis and management of compartment syndromes. *In* AAOS: Symposium on Trauma to the Leg and its Sequela. C. V. Mosby Co., St. Louis, 1981.)

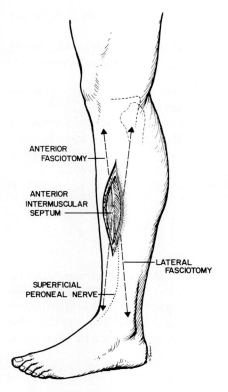

ANTERIOR
FASCIOTOMY

ANTERIOR
INTERMUSCULAR
SEPTUM

LATERAL
FASCIOTOMY

SUPERFICIAL
PERONEAL NERVE

Figure 10–2 Anterolateral incision. Step I: The skin incision utilized to approach the anterior and lateral compartments is placed halfway between the fibular shaft and the tibial crest. (With permission from Mubarak, S. J., and Hargens, A. R.: Diagnosis and management of compartment syndromes. *In* AAOS: Symposium on Trauma to the Leg and its Sequela. C. V. Mosby Co., St. Louis, 1981.)

point, delayed closure at five to seven days without skin grafting is accomplished in nearly all cases. In some cases with very early diagnosis or compartment syndromes initiated by hemorrhage, skin closure following fasciotomy may be possible at the time of initial decompression if pressure measurement is utilized. Certainly, with the limited incision and no skin grafting, a better cosmetic result is obtained.

The disadvantages of the limited incision are twofold. First, on rare occasions when swelling is massive, the skin may actually be a limiting membrane. Second, particularly in the case of a less experienced surgeon, complete fasciotomy may not have been performed if the scissors or fasciotome slip off the fascia. Again, if intraoperative measurement of compartment pressure is utilized, these disadvantages become less important.

Longer skin incisions (20 to 25 cm in length) on both the anterolateral and posteromedial leg should be used when intraoperative tissue pressure measurement is not being used. Also, if the case is delayed and a great deal of swelling is present, longer incisions should be made. The presence of necrotic muscle will frequently require longer incisions for adequate exposure and debridement. Finally, if there is any question in the surgeon's mind regarding the completeness of the fasciotomy, the exposure should be extended for the full length of the compartment. Disadvantages of the more extensive incision are that skin grafting will be required in most cases.

Anterolateral Approach

This is used for an approach to the anterior and/or lateral compartments. The incision is placed halfway between the fibular shaft and the tibial crest. This is approximately over the anterior intermuscular septum dividing the anterior and lateral compartments, and allows easy access to both. The skin edges are undermined proximally and distally to allow for wide exposure of the fascia (Fig. 10–2). Following this, it should be possible to visualize almost the full extent of the compartment fascia. This is an extremely important step when using a more limited incision.

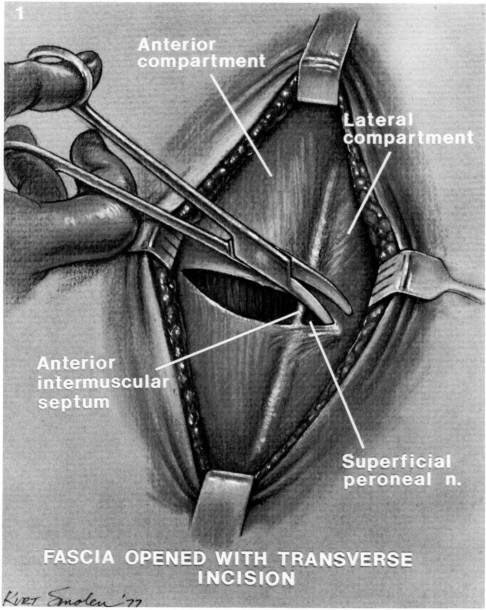

FASCIA OPENED WITH TRANSVERSE INCISION

Figure 10–3 Anterolateral incision. Step II: After undermining the skin edges, a transverse incision is made through the fascia in order to identify the anterior intermuscular septum that separates the anterior compartment from the lateral compartment. (With permission from Mubarak, S. J., and Hargens, A. R.: Diagnosis and management of compartment syndromes. *In* AAOS: Symposium on Trauma to the Leg and its Sequela, C. V. Mosby Co., St. Louis, 1981.)

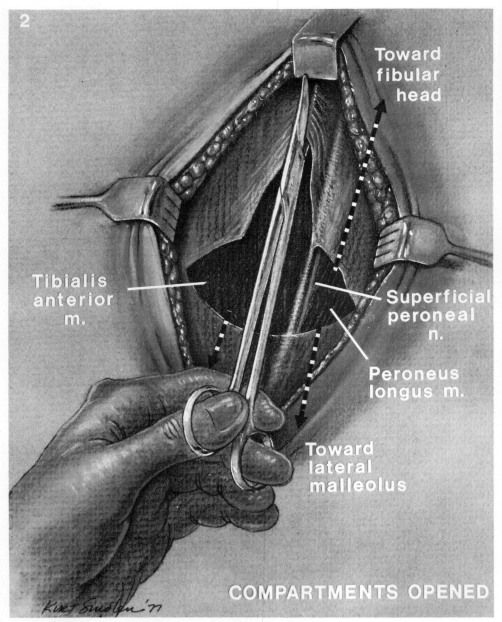

Figure 10–4   Anterolateral incision. Step III: The scissors or fasciotome are pushed in the direction of the great toe distally, and proximally toward the patella, to decompress the anterior compartment. In the lateral compartment they are directed proximally toward the fibular head, and distally toward the lateral malleolus. (With permission from Mubarak, S. J., and Hargens, A. R.: Diagnosis and management of compartment syndromes. *In* AAOS: Symposium on Trauma to the Leg and its Sequela. C. V. Mosby Co., St. Louis, 1981.)

A transverse incision is made just through the fascia in order to identify the anterior intermuscular septum that separates the anterior compartment from the lateral compartment (Fig. 10–3). Identification of this septum is necessary in order to find the superficial peroneal nerve that lies in the lateral compartment next to the septum. Using the 12-inch Metzenbaum scissors, the anterior compartment fascia is opened. Visualization is aided by retraction with right-angled retractors. The scissors are pushed with the tips opened slightly in the direction of the great toe distally, and proximally toward the patella (Fig. 10–4). If there is any question whether the tip of the scissors has strayed from the fascia, the instrument is left in place and a small incision is made over the scissors' tip. If the fasciotomy is incomplete, further release can be performed through this accessory incision.

The lateral compartment fasciotomy is made in line with the fibular shaft. The scissors or fasciotome are directed proximally toward the fibular head and distally toward the lateral malleolus. In this way the fascial incision is posterior to the superficial peroneal nerve. At the completion of this portion of the procedure, both compartments have been widely decompressed, and the superficial peroneal nerve is intact and uninjured (Fig. 10–5).

Posteromedial Approach

This is used for an approach to the superficial and/or deep posterior compartments. This incision is slightly distal to the previous incision and 2 cm posterior to the posterior tibial margin. By making the incision at this location, one avoids injuring the saphenous nerve and vein, which course on the posterior margin of the tibia in this locale (Fig. 10–6). Once again the skin edges are undermined. The saphenous nerve and vein are retracted anteriorly. A transverse fascial incision is made to allow identification of the septum between the deep and superficial posterior compartments (Fig. 10–7). The tendon of the flexor digitorum longus in the deep posterior compartment and the Achilles tendon in the superficial posterior compartment are identified. It is usually easiest to decompress the superficial posterior compartment first. This fasciotomy is extended proximally as far as possible, and then distally behind the medial malleolus (Fig. 10–8). The deep posterior compartment is released

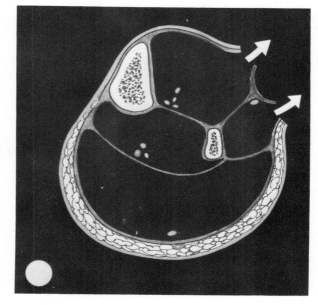

Figure 10–5 Anterolateral incision. Step IV: Cross-section of decompressed anterior and lateral compartments.

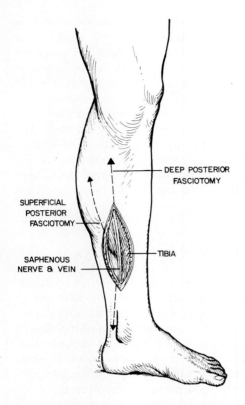

SUPERFICIAL
POSTERIOR
FASCIOTOMY

DEEP POSTERIOR
FASCIOTOMY

SAPHENOUS
NERVE & VEIN

TIBIA

Figure 10–6 Posteromedial incision. Step I: The skin incision used to decompress the superficial and deep posterior compartments is placed 2 cm posterior to the posterior tibial margin. (With permission from Mubarak, S. J., and Hargens, A. R.: Diagnosis and management of compartment syndromes. *In* AAOS: Symposium on Trauma to the Leg and its Sequela. C. V. Mosby Co., St. Louis, 1981.)

distally and then proximally under the soleus bridge. If the soleus attaches to the tibia distally more than halfway, this should be released. Occasionally we have encountered the soleus muscle or fascia extending to near the ankle, completely covering the deeper-lying fascia of the deep posterior compartment. In this case the deep posterior compartment is not visualized until the superficial has been opened and the soleus retracted (Fig. 10–9).

This completes a four-compartment decompression (Fig. 10–10). If intraoperative pressure monitoring has been utilized during this procedure, a final pressure check of each compartment is now performed. In nearly all cases the wounds are packed open and dressings are applied. Usually the leg is immobilized with a posterior splint. On very rare occasions we have closed the skin at the time of the fasciotomy if: (1) the compartment syndrome has been diagnosed and treated early; and (2) wick pressure studies demonstrate that, with skin closure, the pressure does not exceed 10 mm Hg.

If the case is delayed, very little muscle should be debrided at the time of initial decompression. It is very difficult in this situation to differentiate infarcted muscle from ischemic, but recoverable, muscle.

After Care

Approximately five to seven days after fasciotomy the patient is returned to surgery. After this period, and if a more limited skin incision has been made, closure is almost always possible. We have found that vertical mattress suturing (near-far-

far-near technique) is the best for skin closure following fasciotomy (Fig. 10–11). Again, tissue pressure measurement can be of assistance in monitoring the closure.

With large wounds or too much swelling, split-thickness skin grafting will be necessary. Progressive Steri-Strip closure of the wound over a number of days may

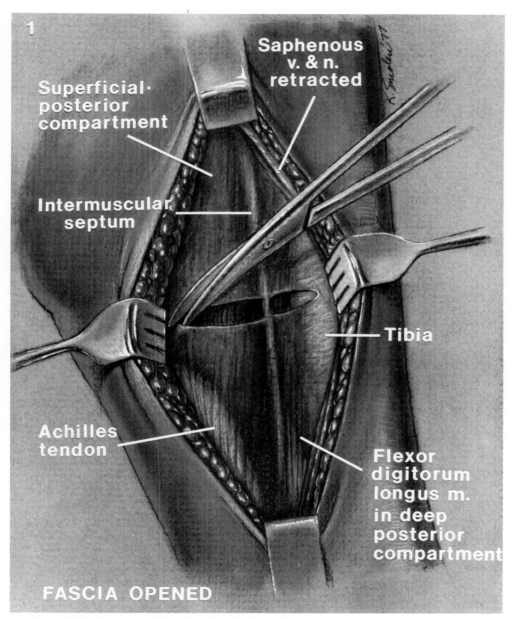

Figure 10–7 Posteromedial incision. Step II: The saphenous nerve and vein are retracted anteriorly. A transverse fascial incision is made to allow identification of the septum between the deep and superficial posterior compartments (With permission from Mubarak, S. J., and Hargens, A. R.: Diagnosis and management of compartment syndromes. *In* AAOS: Symposium on Trauma to the Leg and its Sequela. C. V. Mosby Co., St. Louis, 1981.)

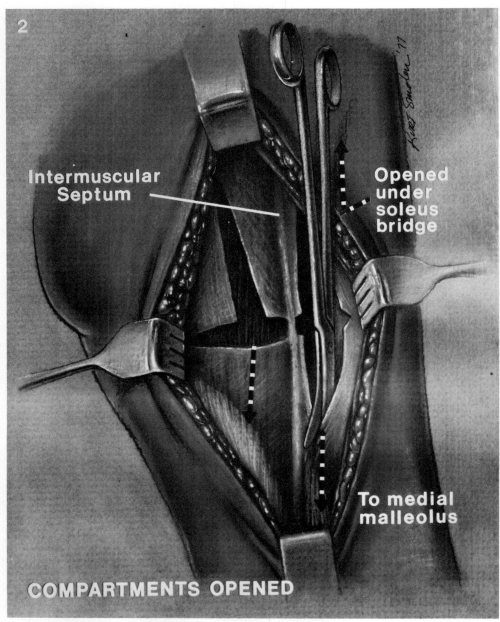

Figure 10–8   Posteromedial incision. Step III: It is easiest to decompress the superficial posterior compartment first. The deep posterior compartment is released distally and then proximally under the soleus bridge. The soleus should be released if it attaches to the tibia more than halfway. (With permission from Mubarak, S. J., and Hargens, A. R.: Diagnosis and management of compartment syndromes. *In* AAOS: Symposium on Trauma to the Leg and its Sequela. C. V. Mosby Co., St. Louis, 1981.)

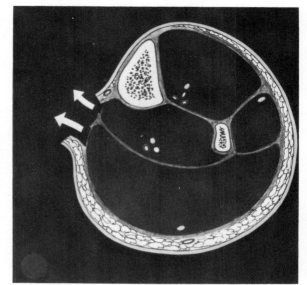

Figure 10–9 Posteromedial incision. Step IV: Cross-section of decompressed superficial and deep posterior compartments.

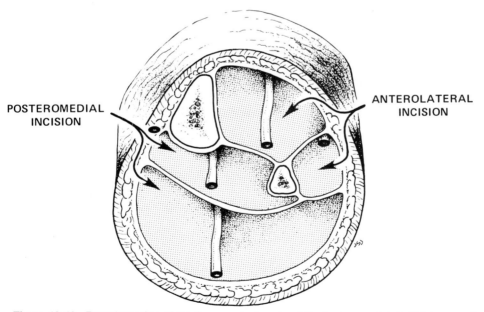

POSTEROMEDIAL INCISION

ANTEROLATERAL INCISION

Figure 10–10 Decompression of the four compartments of the leg is completed. If intraoperative pressure monitoring was utilized during the procedure, a final pressure check of each compartment is now performed. (With permission from Mubarak, S. J., and Owen, C. A.: Double-incision fasciotomy of the leg for decompression of compartment syndromes. J. Bone Joint Surg. 59-A:184–187, 1977.)

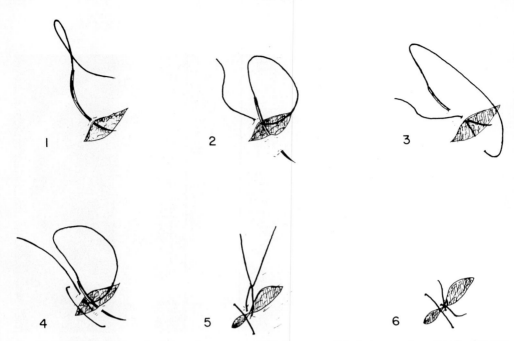

Figure 10–11   Delayed primary closure can usually be accomplished at seven days after fasciotomy, and if more limited skin incisions have been utilized. The vertical mattress suturing technique of near-far-far-near has been found to be quite useful in closing these wounds. The various steps are illustrated.

be helpful to decrease the wound size. This technique, together with meshing of the split-thickness skin graft, is an important adjunct in coverage of the fasciotomy wounds.

If there is necrotic muscle, the wounds are debrided repeatedly once or twice weekly until a satisfactory granulation bed is present. Quantitative bacteria counts have been helpful in deciding when to perform grafting.

Do not overlook the insiduous development of contractures, as even with early diagnosis these may develop in the subacute phase. This may be due to splinting secondary to pain, anterior compartment weakness, or posterior compartment muscle involvement. Posterior splinting of the ankle in the neutral position is mandatory. Figure 10–12 illustrates the short leg-casting technique used to treat the early-developing equinus contracture. With the dorsum of the cast removed, the patient can actively extend the foot and ankle.

TIBIAL FRACTURES AND COMPARTMENT SYNDROMES OF LEG

Occasionally we recommend external fixation of the tibial fracture when this is associated with a compartment syndrome, to facilitate wound care. We generally have used external fixation rather than plates or intramedullary rods. There would appear to be an increased risk of infection when employing internal fixation devices in the face of open wounds and ischemic muscle.

The obvious advantage of immobilizing the fracture is that fasciotomy wound care is facilitated. The major disadvantage of the external fixator or pins and plaster is that mobilization of the skin for delayed primary closure is not as easy, and skin grafting is usually required.

However, when a limited incision is employed with a stable tibial fracture, a long leg cast will be perfectly adequate in immobilizing the fracture and allowing wound care. In our experience this has been the most commonly used technique for treating tibial fractures associated with compartment syndromes.

PROPHYLACTIC FASCIOTOMY OF LEG

Prophylactic fasciotomy is considered for any patient with a substantially high chance of developing a compartment syndrome, e.g.:

Tibial Injuries

Anterior and lateral compartment fasciotomies should be performed on children undergoing tibial osteotomies (Steel et al., 1971; Matsen and Staheli, 1975) or leg lengthening (Mubarak and Carroll, 1979), or when the tibia is used as a donor bone graft site (Mubarak and Carroll, 1979). When debriding an open tibial fracture,

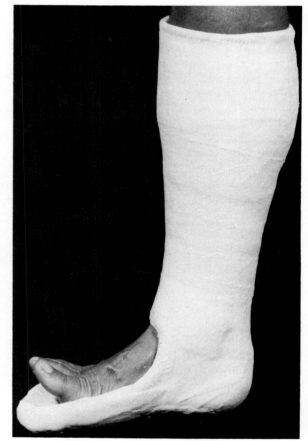

Figure 10–12 To prevent or treat equinus that develops in the subacute phase, the short, leg-casting technique illustrated above is utilized. With the dorsum of the cast removed, the patient can actively extend the foot and ankle. (With permission from Mubarak, S. J., and Hargens, A. R.: Diagnosis and management of compartment syndromes. *In* AAOS: Symposium on Trauma to the Leg and its Sequela. C. V. Mosby Co., St. Louis, 1981.)

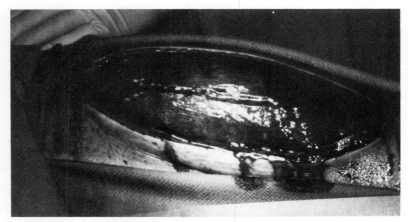

Figure 10–13 Bulging vastus lateralis muscle in a patient who developed multiple compartment syndromes and the crush syndrome from drug overdose-limb compression.

compartments available through the exposed wound should be opened. This should be performed only if the anatomy is not distorted by the fracture and the location of the superficial nerves is apparent. Also, in light of reports by Wiggins (1975) and Wall (1979) on compartment syndromes following Hauser procedures, prophylactic fasciotomy should be strongly considered.

Arterial Injuries

Patients who have sustained an arterial injury or thrombosis, or have had a femoral artery bypass, are especially prone to develop compartment syndromes. Whitesides et al. (1977) have demonstrated that marked swelling and elevated intracompartmental pressure follow six and eight hours of tourniquet ischemia in dogs. In our experience, patients with postischemic compartment syndromes have an especially poor prognosis. This is because the period of ischemia secondary to the arterial injury is additive to the untreated compartment syndrome that results after restitution of the arterial injury. Therefore, if the arterial ischemia lasts for more than six hours, prophylactic, four-compartment fasciotomy of the leg is warranted at the time of arterial repair.

TREATMENT: COMPARTMENT SYNDROMES OF
THIGH

Thigh and buttock areas are involved much less frequently with compartment syndromes than is the leg, probably because of their more expansile compartments. With the increased muscle mass of these areas, the systemic effects of muscle ischemia (i.e., crush syndrome) may predominate, rather than the local effects of the compartment syndrome. Furthermore, the clinical findings will center around increased compartmental pressure and pain with stretch. Sensory deficits are less often observed even with complete myoglobinuric renal failure.

The primary compartments of the thigh are the quadriceps, adductors, and hamstrings. We have noted isolated cases that involved the vastus lateralis muscle but not the other quadriceps (Fig. 10–13). Most of these have been seen in drug overdose-limb compression patients.

The surgical exposure will depend on the areas of involvement. Decompression is performed through a 15- to 20-cm longitudinal skin incision over the involved muscle or compartment. The techniques of fasciotomy are the same as in the leg, using the long Metzenbaum scissors or fasciotome to decompress the involved muscles or compartments (Figs. 10–14, 10–15). Intraoperative monitoring and the postoperative course are identical to those in the plan outlined previously for decompression of the leg.

TREATMENT: COMPARTMENT SYNDROMES OF BUTTOCKS

As with the thigh, involvement of the three gluteal compartments (gluteus maximus, gluteus medius-minimus, and tensor) is primarily seen in drug overdose-limb compression patients. Furthermore, all cases reported (Mubarak and Owen, 1975; Evanski and Waugh, 1977; Owen et al., 1978) have had manifestations of the

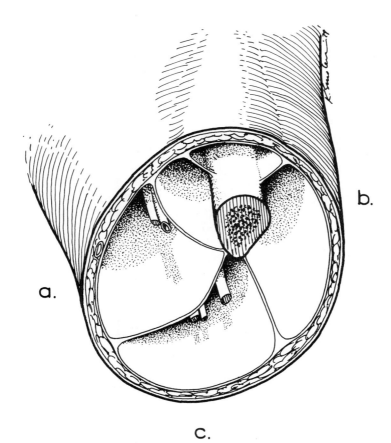

Figure 10–14 Cross-section of the thigh illustrating three approaches to the various anatomic areas. *a*, Approach to the adductor region; *b*, approach to the vastus lateralis and quadriceps; *c*, approach to the hamstrings.

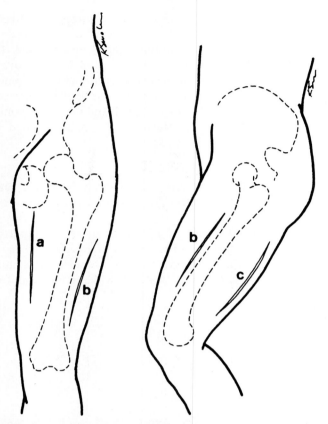

Figure 10–15 Anterior and lateral views of the thigh illustrating three incisions that may be used to approach various compartments of the thigh, as shown in Figure 10–14.

crush syndrome, with myoglobinuric renal failure and markedly elevated creatinine phosphokinase. Sciatic nerve involvement is uncommon with gluteal compartment syndromes, although it has been noted as a complication of excessive bleeding following hip surgery (Fleming et al., 1979).

   We prefer Gibson's posterolateral skin incision (Fig. 10–16). This allows exposure to all three compartments. The fascia superficial to the gluteus maximus is relatively thin and blends with the epimysium, sending septa into the muscle. This forms multiple subdivisions within this large, multipennate muscle belly. To adequately decompress this compartment, multiple incisions in the fascia-epimysium layer are required (Mubarak et al., 1978). Through the same skin incision, the other two compartments of the buttocks (gluteus medius-minimus and tensor) can be decompressed by dividing the iliotibial fascial longitudinally (Owen et al., 1978).

TREATMENT: COMPARTMENT SYNDROMES OF ILIACUS

   The usual etiology of this compartment syndrome is hemorrhage secondary to hemophilia (Brower and Wilde, 1966; Goodfellow et al., 1967), or anticoagulant therapy (Wells and Templeton, 1977) in the iliacus compartment. The typical findings of the iliacus syndrome are a groin mass and severe pain, with the hip held in flexion and slight external rotation. A femoral nerve palsy is usually present.

Unlike the views held regarding any other compartment syndrome, the consensus is to treat this entity nonoperatively (Brower and Wilde, 1966; Goodfellow et al., 1967; Wells and Templeton, 1977). In most cases, the patients are poor surgical risks because of their bleeding diathesis. The aim of therapy is to stop the bleeding and relieve the pain. The appropriate antagonist to treat the bleeding diathesis is given, and the limb is splinted in the position of comfort. Goodfellow et al. (1967) reported 75 per cent complete femoral nerve recovery in 20 cases of the iliacus syndrome caused by hemophilia. Wells and Templeton (1977) reviewed the literature and reported a similar result with 27 cases of femoral neuropathy associated with anticoagulant therapy. Although pressure measurement of the iliacus syndrome has not been reported to clarify this entity, the nonoperative approach seems reasonable in light of the serious risk of further bleeding and the generally good results that attend conservative therapy in these patients.

TREATMENT: COMPARTMENT SYNDROMES OF FOOT/ANKLE

Typically, a portion of the muscle bellies of the peroneus tertius and extensor hallucis longus lie under the extensor retinaculum (crural ligament) of the anterior ankle. Swelling in this area due to an ankle fracture may initiate a minicompartment syndrome. Decompression will be necessary to avoid muscle necrosis or injury to the neurovascular structures of this region.

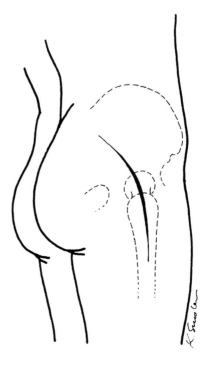

Figure 10–16 Gibson's posterolateral skin incision allows exposure to the three compartments of the buttocks (Gluteus maximus; gluteus medius-minimus; and tensor compartments). (From Crenshaw, A. H. (ed.): Campbell's Operative Orthopaedics, 5th ed. C. V. Mosby Co., St. Louis, 1971.)

The interosseous muscles of the foot are bound in compartments, similar to the interosseous muscles of the hand. Again, with severe soft-tissue injury and subsequent swelling, decompression may be required. For the foot we prefer one or two dorsal, longitudinal incisions over the involved areas. Severe pain and elevated pressure will be the main determinants of the need for this surgery. Involvement of the other compartments of the foot has not been reported.

REFERENCES

Bate, J. T.: A subcutaneous fasciotome. Clin. Orthop. 83:235–236, 1972.

Brower, T. D., and Wilde, A. H.: Femoral neuropathy in hemophilia. J. Bone Joint Surg. 48-A:487–492, 1966.

DeBakey, M. E., and Simeone, F. A.: Battle injuries of the arteries in World War II. An analysis of 2,471 cases. Ann. Surg. 123:534–579, 1946.

Dennis, C.: Disaster following femoral vein ligation for thrombophlebitis; relief by fasciotomy; clinical case of renal impairment following crush injury. Surgery 17:264–269, 1945.

Ernst, C. B., and Kaufer, H.: Fibulectomy-fasciotomy; an important adjunct in the management of lower extremity arterial trauma. J. Trauma 11:365–380, 1971.

Evanski, P. M., and Waugh, T. R.: Gluteal compartment syndrome: case report. J. Trauma 17:323–324, 1977.

Fleming, R. E., Michelsen, C. B., and Stinchfield, F. E.: Sciatic paralysis, a complication of bleeding following hip surgery. J. Bone and Joint Surg. 61-A:37–39, 1979.

Gaspard, D. J., Cohen, J. L., and Gaspar, M. R.: Decompression dermotomy. A limb salvage adjunct. J.A.M.A. 220:831–833, 1972.

Goodfellow, J., Fearn, C. B. D'A., and Mathews, J. M.: Iliacus haematoma, a common complication of haemophilia. J. Bone Joint Surg. 49-B:748–756, 1967.

Jacob, J. E.: Compartment syndrome, a potential course of amputation in battlefield vascular injuries. Int. Surg. 10:542–548, 1974.

Kelly, R. P., and Whitesides, T. E., Jr.: Transfibular route for fasciotomy of the leg. J. Bone Joint Surg. 49-A:1022–1023, 1967.

Matsen, F. A., and Clawson, D. K.: The deep posterior compartmental syndrome of the leg. J. Bone Joint Surg. 57-A:34–39, 1975.

Matsen, F. A., and Krugmire, R. B.: Compartment syndromes. Surg. Gynecol. Obstet. 147:943–949, 1978.

Matsen, F. A., and Staheli, L. T.: Neurovascular complications following tibial osteotomy in children. A case report. Clin. Orthop. 110:210–214, 1975.

Mozes, M., Ramon, Y., and Jahr, J.: The anterior tibial syndrome. J. Bone Joint Surg. 44-A:730–736, 1962.

Mubarak, S. J., and Carroll, N. C.: Volkmann's contracture in children; aetiology and prevention. J. Bone Joint Surg. 61-B:285–293, 1979.

Mubarak, S. J., and Owen, C. A.: Compartment syndrome and its relation to the crush syndrome; a spectrum of disease. Clin. Orthop. 113:81–89, 1975.

Mubarak, S. J., and Owen, C. A.: Double incision fasciotomy of the leg for decompression in compartment syndromes. J. Bone Joint Surg. 59-A:184–187, 1977.

Mubarak, S. J., Owen, C. A., Hargens, A. R., Garetto, L. P., and Akeson, W. H.: Acute compartment syndromes; diagnosis and treatment with the aid of the wick catheter. J. Bone Joint Surg. 60-A:1091–1095, 1978.

Owen, C. A., Woody, P. R., Mubarak, S. J., and Hargens, A. R.: Gluteal compartment syndromes; a report of three cases and management utilizing the wick catheter. Clin. Orthop. 132:57–60, 1978.

Patman, R. D.: Compartmental syndromes in peripheral vascular surgery. Arch. Surg. 101:663–670, 1970.

Patman, R. D., and Thompson, J. E.: Fasciotomy in peripheral vascular surgery. Arch. Surg. 101:663–670, 1970.

Rosato, F. E., Barier, C. F., Roberts, B, and Danielson, G. K.: Subcutaneous fasciotomy, description of a new technique and instrument. Surgery 59:383, 1966.

Seddon, H. J.: Volkmann's ischaemia in the lower limb. J. Bone Joint Surg. 48-B:627–636, 1966.

Sirbu, A. B., Murphy, M. J., and White, A. S.: Soft tissue complications of fracture of the leg. Calif. West. Med. 60:53–56, 1944.

Steel, H. H., Sandrow, R. E., and Sullivan, P. D.: Complications of tibial osteotomy in children for genu varum or valgum. J. Bone Joint Surg. 53-A:1629–1635, 1971.

Wall, J. J.: Compartment syndrome as a complication of the Hauser procedure. J. Bone Joint Surg. 61-A:185–191, 1979.

Wells, J., and Templeton, J.: Femoral neuropathy associated with anticoagulant therapy. Clin. Orthop. 124:155–160, 1977.

Whitesides, T. E., Jr., Hirada, H., and Morimoto, K.: Compartment syndromes and the role of fasciotomy, its parameters and techniques. Am. Acad. Orthop. Surg., Instructional Course Lectures 26:179–194, 1977.

Wiggins, H. E.: The anterior tibial compartment syndrome. A complication of the Hauser technique. Clin. Orthop. 113:90–94, 1975.

Willhoite, D. R., and Moll, J. H.: Early recognition of impending Volkmann's ischemia in the lower extremity. Arch. Surg. 100:11–16, 1970.

Chapter Eleven

THE CRUSH SYNDROME

Charles A. Owen, M.D.

The crush syndrome is the systemic result of muscle necrosis consisting of myoglobinuria, third-space fluid loss, shock, acidosis, hyperkalemia, and renal failure.

HISTORY

Bywaters and Beall in 1941 reported cases of civilian casualties during the London blitz, with crush injuries to the extremities from bombing debris, who manifested this clinical picture (Fig. 11–1). This appears to be the first report of this syndrome in the English literature. As more cases arose, it became apparent that they represented a distinct clinical entity with a common etiologic factor of muscle necrosis. The term "crush syndrome" was suggested by the Hammersmith Hospital group, and eventually was adopted into general use (Bywaters and McMichael, 1953).

After the war these English workers reviewed the German literature and found a description of the syndrome by Frankenthal (1916), who reported three cases. Weiting (1918) described a case treated by multiple incisions. Minami (1923) reviewed the syndrome and suggested the possibility of the involvement of myoglobin, which had just been differentiated from hemoglobin. The official German War Surgery Handbook, published in 1922, described 126 cases (Kayser, 1922). Surprisingly, there is no record in the English literature following World War I of any recognition of the syndrome, although several case reports have retrospectively been diagnosed as such. Perhaps the first description of muscle necrosis associated with coma was by Larrey (1812), who had opportunity to examine several cases of soldiers poisoned by carbon monoxide. He reported skin and muscle necrosis in areas of pressure (Howse and Seddon, 1966).

Subsequent to the report of Bywaters and Beall (1941), considerable interest in the problem was aroused. Later in the same year, myoglobin was isolated from the urine of crush syndrome cases, establishing beyond doubt the association of the renal failure with muscle damage (Bywaters et al., 1941). Both clinical and experimental studies correlated the extent of renal failure with the amount of muscle damage. Considerable work on renal failure in both England and the United States

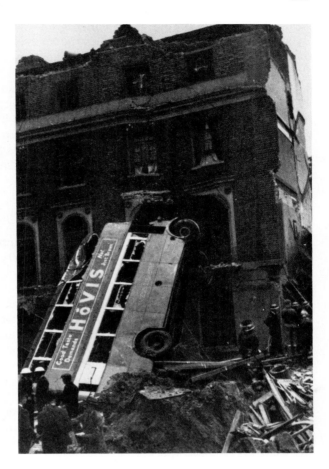

Figure 11–1 London street scene. Sept. 8, 1940. (From Fleming, P.: Invasion, 1940. Rupert Hart-Davis, London, 1957.)

during World War II suggested that acidosis and decreased renal blood flow, secondary to shock, might also be important factors in the renal problems in these patients.

Understandably, interest in the crush syndrome waned somewhat after the cessation of hostilities and bombing in 1945. In 1953, however, Gordon and Newman reported a case without massive trauma, but following prolonged anesthesia in the knee-chest position. Howse and Seddon (1966) reported four cases of ischemic limb contracture secondary to carbon monoxide and barbiturate overdose, but none of these patients had documented renal failure. Subsequently, many reports have appeared dealing with prolonged limb compression, myoglobinuria, and renal impairment in drug overdose patients (Linton et al., 1968; Schreiber et al., 1971, 1972; Penn et al., 1972; Dolich and Aiache, 1973).

ETIOLOGY

Although the initial recognition and description of this syndrome concerned patients whose extremities were compressed by external debris, this mechanism is now unusual. Isolated cases continue to appear, however, and in 1968 Bentley reported three cases occurring in patients who were buried in coal mine accidents. Recognition of the problems caused by the knee-chest position for spine surgery has made this an uncommon cause (Gordon and Newman, 1953; Keim and Weinstein, 1970) (Fig. 11–3).

Currently, however, by far the most common underlying etiology is drug overdose, with compression of the individual's extremities by his own torso or head. Drugs inducing long periods of coma, such as the barbiturates or heroin, are most commonly involved. In our experience, there appears to be a recent decrease in the incidence of drug-induced crush syndrome, perhaps because of a current preference for hallucinogenic drugs that do not tend to cause long periods of immobility.

PATHOGENESIS

The crush syndrome is characterized by myoglobinuric renal failure, initiated by prolonged compression of skeletal muscle by debris or the victim's own body. Myoglobinuria is the result of the release of myoglobin from muscle tissue, and may or may not be associated with renal failure. Many etiologies of myoglobinuria other than limb compression have been described, including hereditary disease such as McArdle's, prolonged exercise in normal individuals, convulsions, malignant hyperthermia, influenza, and toxins such as snake venom (Rowland and Penn, 1972; Cunningham et al., 1979). Myoglobin, a protein synthesized in muscle, is important in oxygen transport and storage, and is found in high concentrations in type I oxidative fibers. Its appearance in the urine probably requires at least 200 mg of damaged muscle (Berenbaum et al., 1953).

Although a relationship between prolonged compression of skeletal muscle and myoglobinuria has been well established in the voluminous literature since 1941, the exact pathogenesis of the crush syndrome has remained in doubt. There is agreement that prolonged limb compression can produce sufficient rhabdomyolysis to produce myoglobinuria, but the exact cause of the muscle ischemia and necrosis has remained controversial. Early reports of the crush syndrome involved victims who were buried under massive debris, and the production of muscle necrosis by direct pressure was easy to understand. The recognition of a crush syndrome secondary to prolonged immobility from drug overdose or surgical knee-chest position raised new questions about the etiology of the muscle necrosis. Although most authors continued to believe that muscle damage resulted from direct pressure on the extremity by the patient's own head or torso, many other causes were suggested. Some believed that heroin or barbiturates have a direct myotoxic effect (Richter et al., 1971; Rowland and Penn, 1972; Klock and Sexton, 1973), and others suggested that the hypoxemia alone resulting from the systemic effects of drug overdose is sufficient to cause myonecrosis (Graham, 1962). Occlusion of the major arterial inflow by direct pressure has also been implicated (Keim and Weinstein, 1970; Penn et al., 1972).

Our early studies with the wick catheter in a small number of normal individuals demonstrated significantly elevated intramuscular pressures in extremities subjected to compression by the person's own head or torso. We hypothesized, therefore, that the drug overdose-induced crush syndrome was initiated by localized muscle and capillary necrosis from ischemia produced by compression from the patient's own head or torso. We verified this hypothesis by measuring pressures

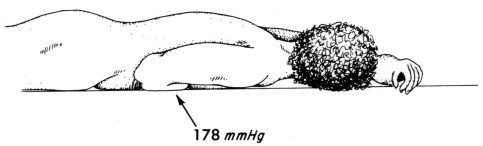

178 *mmHg*

Figure 11–2   Rib-cage compression of forearm (pressure range 100 to 225 mm Hg; mean 178 mm Hg).

within the muscles of extremities subjected to such compression (Owen et al., 1979). Wick catheters were inserted into ten flexor compartments of forearm muscles and ten anterior tibial compartment muscles in 17 normal volunteers, who were then placed in the positions in which drug overdose victims are commonly found. With continuous monitoring of the intramuscular pressure, the individual's position was varied slightly until a maximal wick pressure was recorded.

The mean maximal pressures obtained on a hard surface are shown in Figures 11–2 to 11–6. A softer surface (2.5-cm foam padding) decreased the mean maximum an average 16 per cent in the leg and 23 per cent in the forearm. Pressures fell progressively from the point of maximal compression, but remained significantly elevated in an area 6 to 8 cm in diameter. Pulses distal to the compression site were undiminished to palpation in all positions except rib cage-forearm (Fig. 11–2) and knee-chest (Fig. 11–3). The radial pulse disappeared in two of ten individuals and diminished in three with rib cage compression, and in the knee-chest position pedal pulses were consistently diminished or obliterated when knee or hip flexion exceeded 130 degrees.

Eighty per cent of the pressures were 50 mm Hg or more, and in only two instances were pressures on hard surfac s less than 30 mm Hg. We believe that these studies clearly demonstrate that compression of limb musculature by a person's own body can produce sufficient pressure in almost all instances to cause muscle

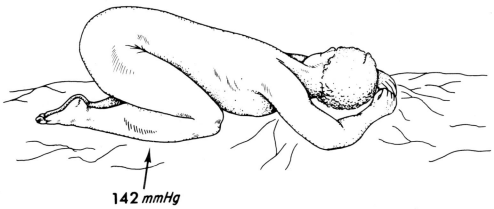

142 *mmHg*

Figure 11–3   Surgical knee-chest position with compression of anterior compartment of leg (pressure range 105 to 240 mm Hg; mean 142 mm Hg).

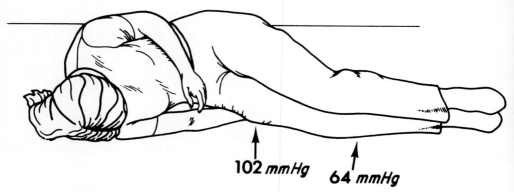

102 *mmHg*   64 *mmHg*

Figure 11–4   Trunk compression of forearm (pressure range 30 to 160 mm Hg; mean 102 mm Hg) and leg (pressure range 29 to 160 mm Hg; mean 64 mm Hg).

ischemia by local obstruction to the circulation and, if maintained for a sufficient period, will cause necrosis of muscle and capillary wall.

Clinical findings also support the concept of a local tamponade of circulation. Many authors have reported a correlation between skin changes (erythema and so-called "barb blisters") and the position of immobilization (Orizaga et al., 1967; Weeks, 1968; Conner, 1971; Schreiber et al., 1972; Dolich and Aiache, 1973; Kaufer et al., 1974; Mubarak and Owen, 1975). These skin changes also are undoubtedly due to ischemia secondary to pressure. Furthermore, surgical exploration has frequently demonstrated localized muscle ischemia corresponding to the areas of skin changes that was not related to arterial supply (Howse and Seddon, 1966; Linton et al., 1968;

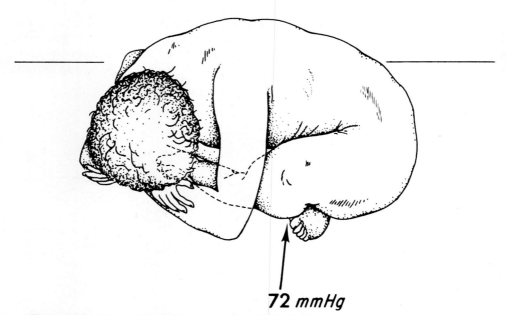

72 *mmHg*

Figure 11–5   Yoga position with compression of the leg by feet (pressure range 49 to 125 mm Hg; mean 72 mm Hg).

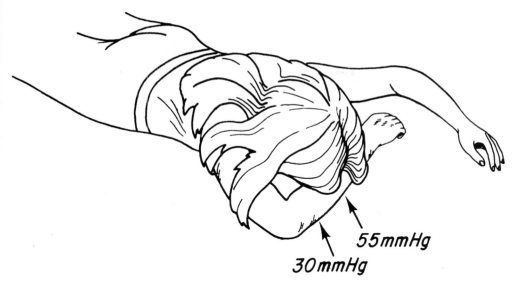

Figure 11–6 Head compression of forearm (pressure range 26 to 75 mm Hg; mean 55 mm Hg).

Weeks, 1968; Conner, 1971; Penn et al., 1972; Schreiber et al., 1972; Dolich and Aiache, 1973; Kaufer et al., 1974; Mubarak and Owen, 1975).

Although other factors such as hypoxemia, metabolic acidosis, hypothermia, hypovolemic shock, or (rarely) vascular occlusion may be contributory, the primary factor is localized muscle and capillary ischemia secondary to pressure tamponade. In some patients the process may end at this stage, with only a localized area of muscle necrosis and some myoglobinuria. In others with more extensive local injury, however, sufficient edema may be produced to initiate a compartment syndrome with its self-perpetuating edema-ischemia cycle (Fig. 11–7). Whether the systemic manifestations of the full-blown crush syndrome appear depends on the amount of muscle that is infarcted. In a review of 11 cases of prolonged limb compression, we were able to correlate the severity of the crush syndrome with the number of compartments involved (Mubarak and Owen, 1975). We believe that there is a relationship between a compartment syndrome and the crush syndrome, representing a spectrum of disease from single compartment involvement without renal failure to multiple compartment involvement with renal failure.

Once a significant amount of muscle has become infarcted, the systemic manifestations appear. Loss of functional integrity of the sarcolemma results in intracellular edema, and this, coupled with interstitial edema resulting from capillary ischemic damage, may produce significant third-space loss. In the absence of intravascular fluid replacement, hypovolemia with hypotension or shock may result. Muscle cellular breakdown results in the release of myoglobin into the circulation.

The exact pathogenesis of myoglobinuric renal failure is not completely understood. Myoglobin is deposited in the distal convoluted tubule, which ultimately causes occlusion. This may precipitate renal failure, but other factors such as renal tubular anoxia secondary to hypotension appear to be contributory.

Potassium released from damaged muscle cells is not excreted in the presence of renal failure, and hyperkalemia may produce cardiac arrhythmias. For a more

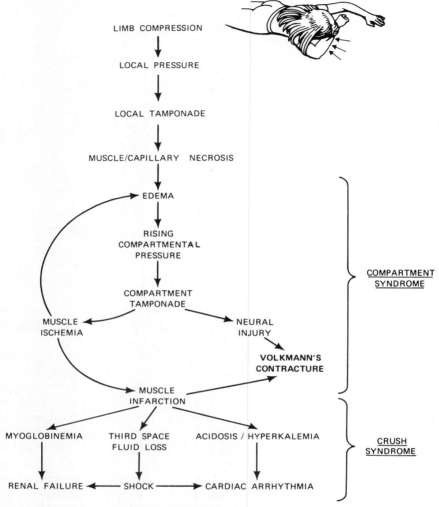

Figure 11–7 Pathogenesis of the prolonged limb compression-compartment syndrome-crush syndrome. (With permission from Owen, C. A., et al.: Intramuscular pressures with limb compression. N. Engl. J. Med. 300:1169–1172, 1979.)

complete review of myoglobinuria and acute renal failure, the reader is referred to several excellent sources (Rowland and Penn, 1972; Schrier, 1979).

CLINICAL PRESENTATION

History

The history is usually obvious in victims buried under debris, either in wartime or civilian life, such as in coal-mining accidents (Figs. 11–8, 11–9). In some cases, almost the entire body other than the head has been buried. The duration of burial under debris has usually been more than six hours.

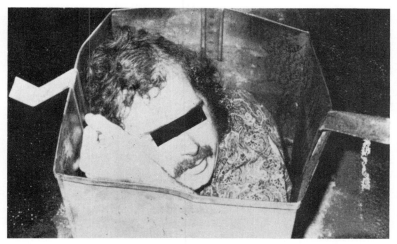

Figure 11–8 Case 1. Unusual civilian etiology of limb compression in which a burglar became wedged in a vent for 4½ hours. The patient was brought to the hospital with bilateral forearm compartment syndromes and a stage II crush syndrome. Immediate fasciotomy resulted in normal limbs. (With permission from Mubarak, S. J., and Owen, C. A.: Compartmental syndrome and its relation to the crush syndrome: a spectrum of disease. Clin. Orthop. 113:81–89, 1975.)

In the more commonly seen drug overdose patients today, an accurate history is often difficult or impossible to obtain upon admission. Frequently, there is no witness, and the narcotizing agent and duration of immobility may be impossible to determine immediately. The most common drugs have been the barbiturates, particularly secobarbital. Heroin also is frequently involved. The estimated duration of immobility in our study of 11 patients was four to 48 hours, averaging approximately 12 hours.

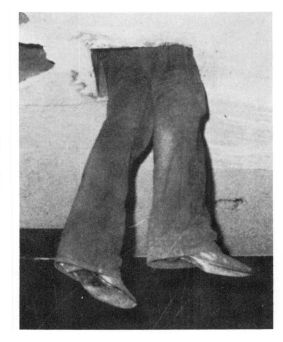

Figure 11–9 Case 1. Looking up at ceiling vent, showing burglar hanging by compressed forearms. (With permission from Mubarak, S. J., and Owen, C. A.: Compartmental syndrome and its relation to the crush syndrome: a spectrum of disease. Clin. Orthop. 113:81–89, 1975.)

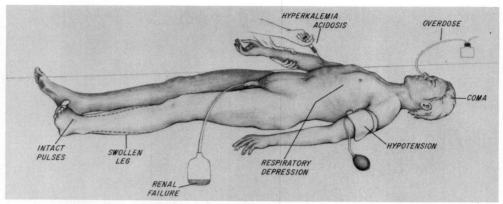

Figure 11–10 Typical findings soon after hospital admission in a drug overdose patient sustaining limb compression with resulting crush syndrome (stage III). (With permission from Mubarak, S. J., and Owen, C. A.: Compartmental syndrome and its relation to the crush syndrome: a spectrum of disease. Clin. Orthop. 113:81–89, 1975.)

Examination

The major systemic problems seen in drug overdose-limb compression patients are usually quite obvious. Many exhibit some degree of obtundation or coma, with respiratory depression secondary to the narcotizing drugs. They may be in shock secondary to hypovolemia from third-space fluid loss and dehydration. Urine output may be low or absent (Fig. 11–10).

These overwhelming medical problems, requiring emergency resuscitative measures, frequently divert attention from the compressed limb. Unless there is a high degree of suspicion, the extremities may not be carefully examined. There may be localized skin pressure changes with erythema, bullae, or vesicles (Fig. 11–11). There may be only minimal swelling of the extremities on the initial examination because of dehydration and peripheral vasoconstriction secondary to shock. As these problems are corrected by fluid replacement, third-space loss into the involved extremities may occur, producing swelling that may be rather massive. Rarely, the deltoid and gluteal compartments may be involved (Mubarak et al., 1978; Owen et al., 1978).

The diagnosis of a compartment syndrome on clinical grounds is difficult if patients are either uncooperative, obtunded, or comatose. One cannot then elicit the usual important clinical findings that are dependent on patient response, e.g., pain with muscle stretch, sensory deficit, or motor weakness. The diagnosis must therefore be *suspected* simply on the history of prolonged immobilization and the finding of a swollen extremity, and *confirmed* by other means, namely, intracompartmental pressure measurement.

Laboratory

Laboratory studies for the most part reflect the degree of systemic manifestation of the crush syndrome. Muscle injury is reflected in increased enzyme levels,

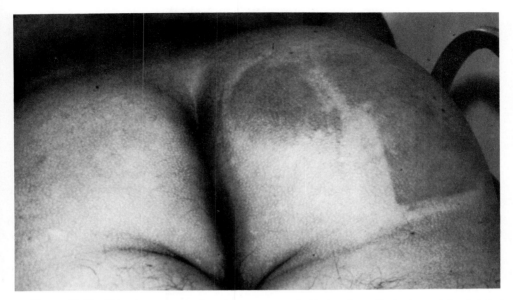

Figure 11–11 Skin changes secondary to pressure on buttocks of a patient who sustained gluteal compartment syndrome and a crush syndrome.

including aldolase, SGOT, LDH, CPK.* The CPK is usually elevated over 10,000 international units (IU). Myoglobin may be identified in the urine by a variety of laboratory methods, from spectrophotometry to immunoelectrophoresis. Results of these tests, however, are not rapidly received from the laboratory, and a presumptive diagnosis of myoglobinuria may be made by a positive benzidine test (urine dipstick) for occult blood in the absence of red blood cells on microscopic examination (Table 11–1).

The white blood count and hematocrit may be elevated because of hemoconcentration secondary to third-space fluid loss. Creatinine and blood urea nitrogen levels

---

* SGOT = serum glutamic oxaloacetic transaminase; LDH = lactic dehydrogenase; CPK = creatine phosphokinase.

Table 11–1 TYPICAL URINALYSIS IN PATIENT WITH THE CRUSH SYNDROME AND MYOGLOBINURIA (OCCULT BLOOD: POSITIVE AND RBC = 0)

Macroscopic			Microscopic		
Color	—	Reddish-brown	RBC	—	0
Appearance	—	Clear	WBC	—	Rare
Specific Gravity	—	1.008	Renal Cells	—	0
pH	—	7.0	Bacteria	—	0
Protein	—	2+	Squamous Epithelium	—	Few
Glucose	—	Negative	Mucous Threads	—	0
Ketones	—	Negative	Crystals	—	0
Occult Blood	—	Large Amount (Positive)	Casts	—	0

reflect the severity of the renal failure. Although large amounts of potassium may be released from injured muscle cells, normal kidneys are able to excrete the extra potassium, and hyperkalemia is usually seen only in the presence of associated renal failure.

DIAGNOSIS

As previously noted, the diagnosis of compartment syndrome in drug overdose-limb compression patients may be impossible on clinical grounds because they may be uncooperative, obtunded, or comatose. The valuable clinical signs of ischemia-muscle stretch pain, sensory deficit, or motor weakness therefore are unobtainable or unreliable. The only physical finding may be a swollen, tense extremity. In our review of the 11 cases of prolonged limb compression, the etiology of the swollen limbs on admission was incorrectly attributed to fracture, superficial thrombophlebitis, deep vein thrombosis, or cellulitis in almost half the cases.

Because of the absence of good clinical findings in most of these cases, we consider this situation to be an absolute indication for intracompartmental pressure measurement as an objective criterion for decompressive fasciotomy.

CLASSIFICATION

On the basis of our review of 11 cases of prolonged limb compression, we devised a classification of the compartment syndrome-crush syndrome spectrum of diseases (Mubarak and Owen, 1975).

Stage I.   This stage of the crush syndrome shows elevation of muscle enzymes, with CPK usually greater than 10,000 IU and myoglobinuria. Essentially, any compartment syndrome that is not decompressed early will produce these changes.

Stage II.   This stage shows more marked enzyme elevations, with CPK greater than 20,000 IU, myoglobinura, and elevation of serum creatinine and BUN, without oliguria. On admission these patients are frequently hypotensive from third-spacing of fluid into the extremity.

Stage III.   This stage demonstrates the full picture of the crush syndrome, with oliguria, shock, metabolic acidosis, hyperkalemia, and possible cardiac arrhythmias.

TREATMENT

The sometimes overwhelming medical problems of coma, hypovolemic shock, respiratory depression, and renal failure quite appropriately command immediate attention. Ventilatory support may be necessary. Hypovolemic shock should be treated with rapid replacement of intravascular fluid volume by crystalloid. The patients have sustained plasma, not blood, loss, and are hemoconcentrated. Whole blood therefore should not be used for replacement. In the face of renal failure, fluid overload must be carefully avoided, and central venous pressure or pulmonary arterial pressures should be monitored. Diuretics may be used in the treatment of oliguria. Dialysis may be required. The reader is referred to the report of Weeks (1968) for the specific details of medical management of the crush syndrome.

Successful treatment of the involved extremities depends on prompt diagnosis. A high index of suspicion and the finding of swollen extremities should lead to immediate orthopedic consultation, and in the presence of confusing clinical signs, intracompartmental pressure should be measured. Without benefit of clinical signs to follow progression, we believe that fasciotomy should be performed promptly if pressures exceed 30 mm Hg. Fasciotomy is the only known method of interrupting the self-perpetuating edema-ischemia cycle once critical pressures have been exceeded.

There sometimes is reluctance to subject the medically ill patient to surgical procedures, but it should be emphasized that fasciotomies can usually be performed with a very minimal general, or even local, anesthesia in the narcotized patient. Furthermore, we believe that decompression by fasciotomy is important to diminish the systemic effects of the crush syndrome by preventing further muscle necrosis, as well as to decrease the local compartment sequelae. It is our opinion, therefore, that if intracompartmental pressures are elevated, fasciotomy should be performed even if there is little chance of limb salvage.

Fasciotomies for compartment syndromes secondary to prolonged limb compression should be done through incisions long enough to inspect all of the compartment musculature adequately. Necrotic muscle is not infrequently encountered at the time of fasciotomy in these patients, in contrast to the more usual etiologies in which it is rare to see clearly necrotic muscle at the time of fasciotomy. The reasons for this are twofold. First, as clarified by our experimental studies, the initiating problem is one of localized pressure causing necrosis of muscle. By the time the patient reaches the hospital, this muscle may already have infarcted sufficiently to be demarcated. Second, delayed diagnosis of the superimposed compartment syndrome is very common because of the overwhelming medical problems and the lack of clinical signs and symptoms. Fasciotomy, therefore, may be delayed to a point at which more generalized muscle necrosis from the compartment syndrome has proceeded to demarcation.

The wounds should be left open initially and reinspected at five to seven days, or sooner if problems are anticipated or suspected. Multiple trips to the operating room may be necessary for debridement of further necrotic tissue. Excision of any necrotic muscle will help to prevent scar formation and allow the remaining muscle to function maximally. If the diagnosis has been made promptly, delayed primary wound closure is usually possible at five to seven days. If closure is delayed because of the need for multiple debridements, or if skin edges cannot be approximated, a mesh, split-thickness skin graft may be used.

RESULTS

The results of treatment of the medical aspects of the crush syndrome are generally excellent. Drug-induced coma, respiratory depression, hypovolemic shock, and myoglobinuric renal failure are problems that generally are rapidly diagnosed and treated by standard methods. There were no deaths in our 16 cases of the crush syndrome secondary to prolonged limb compression between 1970 and 1976.

In contrast to the excellent success rate with the systemic problem, severe limb residuals have been common. In the 11 patients treated at University Hospital in San Diego from 1970 to 1973, prior to the development of the wick catheter, the limb results were disastrous. There was a satisfactory outcome in only three of 15 involved limbs. All of these had early fasciotomy. Ten extremities had severe residual contractures. Overall, 80 per cent of the limbs and 80 per cent of the patients had significant residual contracture and nerve deficit (Mubarak and Owen, 1975).

The five patients seen between 1974 and 1976 following the development of the wick catheter had somewhat better overall results (Figs. 11–12 to 11–17). This improvement probably is not entirely attributable to the use of the wick catheter, but to an overall increased awareness of the problem. Three of these five cases had normal outcomes following fasciotomy. One patient had mild residual gluteus medius atrophy and very slight sciatic nerve sensory deficit. The other patient with residual was diagnosed and treated by fasciotomy immediately after admission, but a severe Volkmann's contracture of the forearm still developed. This latter case illustrates the fact that drug-induced coma may so delay admission to the hospital that irreversible damage has already occurred (Mubarak et al., 1978).

It is important to re-emphasize that there may be three reasons for delay in treatment of the compartment syndromes. First, there is usually a delay in hospitalizaton in the drug overdose patient because of his comatose condition. Second, following admission, there may be a delay in diagnosis owing to a preoccupation with other severe medical problems and the absence of the usual clinical signs and symptoms of a compartment syndrome in the comatose patient. Finally, delay in surgical decompression may occur even after accurate diagnosis because of a reluctance to operate upon a seriously ill patient, and the failure to understand the significance of decompression in treating both the compartment syndrome and the crush syndrome.

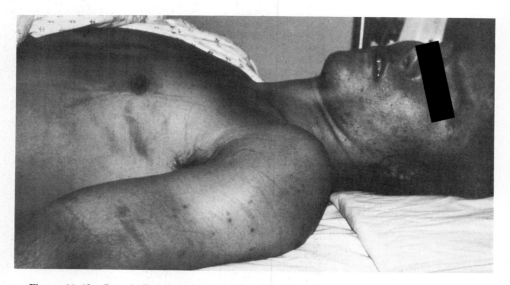

Figure 11–12   Case 2. Twenty-one year old male who overdosed on heroin. He presented to the hospital obtunded, and subsequently required a respirator. He also needed peritoneal dialysis for the resulting crush syndrome and renal failure. The left shoulder and arm were markedly swollen, and skin pressure sores were present on the chest.

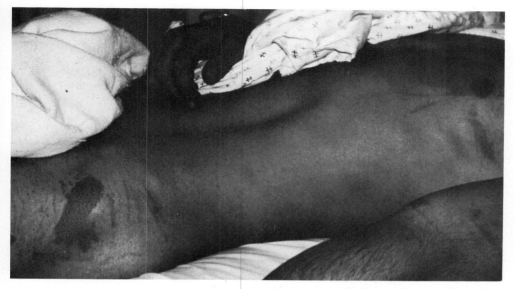

Figure 11–13   Case 2. The pressure areas on the left chest and left thigh are illustrated.

Figure 11–14   Case 2. Wick catheter pressure measurements demonstrate markedly elevated pressures in the deltoid, with only moderately elevated pressures in the biceps (21 mm Hg). The volar forearm pressure was 3 mm Hg.

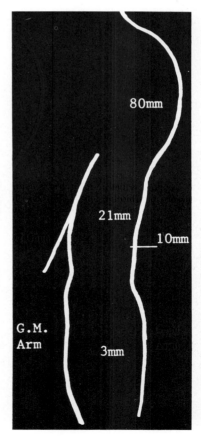

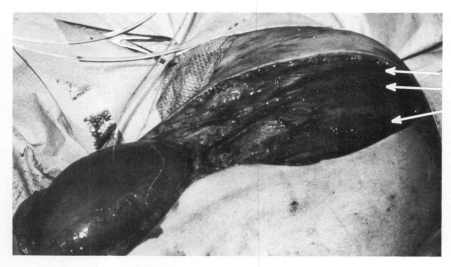

Figure 11–15 Case 2. Intraoperative photo of this patient's anterior left deltoid and biceps. Note that the epimysium and fascia of the deltoid are one, and that multiple epimysial-fascial incisions are required *(see arrows)* to decompress this muscle compartment.

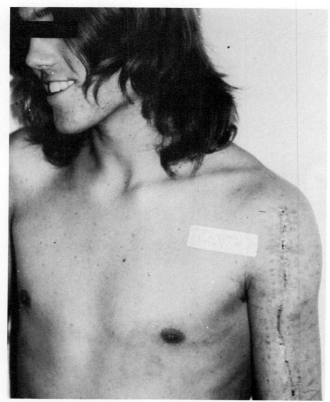

Figure 11–16 Case 2. The patient underwent delayed primary closure at one week. This photo was obtained one month after surgical decompression. Renal function was normal and the fasciotomy wound was well healed.

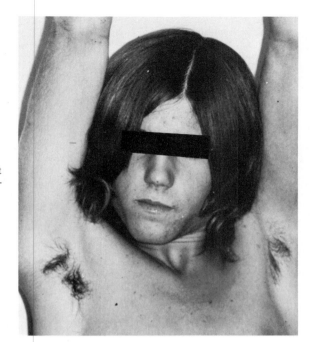

Figure 11–17 Case 2. The patient had full range of motion without contractures or neurologic deficit.

REFERENCES

Bentley, G., and Jeffreys, T. E.: The crush syndrome in coal miners. J. Bone Joint Surg. 50-B:588–594, 1968.

Berenbaum, M. C., Birch, C. A., and Moreland, J. D.: Paroxysmal myoglobinuria. Lancet 1:892–895, 1953.

Bywaters, E. G. L., and Beall, D.: Crush injuries with impairment of renal function. Br. Med. J. 1:427–432, 1941.

Bywaters, E. G. L., Delory, G. E., Remington, C., and Smiles, J.: Myohaemoglobin in urine of air raid casualties with crushing injury. Biochem. J. 35:1164–1168, 1941.

Bywaters, E. G. L., and McMichael, J.: Crush syndrome. In Cope, Z. (ed.): History of the Second World War: Surgery. H. M. Stationery Office, London, 1953, pp. 673–686.

Conner, A. N.: Prolonged external pressure as a cause of ischaemic contracture. J. Bone Joint Surg. 53-B:118–122, 1971.

Cunningham, E., Kohli, R., and Venuto, R. C.: Influenza-associated myoglobinuric renal failure. J.A.M.A. 242:2428–2429, 1979.

Dolich, B. H., and Aiache, A. E.: Drug-induced coma: a cause of the crush syndrome and ischemic contracture. J. Trauma 13:223–228, 1973.

Frankenthal, L.: Uber Verschüttungen. Virchows Arch. 222:332, 1916.

Gordon, B. S., and Newman, W.: Lower nephron syndrome following prolonged knee-chest position. J. Bone Joint Surg. 35-A:764–768, 1953.

Graham, J. D.: The Diagnosis and Treatment of Acute Poisoning. Oxford University Press, London, 1962.

Howse, A. J. G., and Seddon, H.: Ischaemic contracture of muscle associated with carbon monoxide and barbiturate poisoning. Br. Med. J. 1:192–195, 1966.

Kaufer, H., Spengler, D. M., Noyes, F. R., and Louis, D. S.: Orthopaedic implication of the drug subculture. J. Trauma 14:853–867, 1974.

Kayser, F. F. O.: Von Schjerning's Handbuch der Artzlichen Erfahrungen im Weltkriege. Chirugie 36, Leipzig 1, 1922.

Keim, H. A., and Weinstein, J. D.: Acute renal failure: a complication of spine fusion in the tuck position. J. Bone Joint Surg. 52-A:1248–1250, 1970.

Klock, J. C., and Sexton, M. J.: Rhabdomyolysis and acute myoglobinuric renal failure following heroin use. Calif. Med. 119:5–8, 1973.

Linton, A. L., Adams, J. H., and Lawson, D. H.: Muscle necrosis and renal failure in carbon monoxide poisoning. Postgrad. Med. J. 44:338–341, 1968.

Minami, S.: Uber Nierenveränderungen nach Verschüttung. Virchows Arch. 245:247, 1923.

Mubarak, S. J., and Owen, C. A.: Compartmental syndrome and its relation to the crush syndrome: a spectrum of disease. Clin. Orthop. 113:81–89, 1975.

Mubarak, S. J., Owen, C. A., Hargens, A. R., Garetto, L. P., and Akeson, W. H.: Acute compartment syndromes: diagnosis and treatment with the aid of the wick catheter. J. Bone Joint Surg. 60-A:1091–1095, 1978.

Orizaga, M., Ducharme, F. A., Campbell, J. S., and Embree, G. H.: Muscle infarction and Volkmann's contracture following carbon monoxide poisoning. J. Bone Joint Surg. 49-A:965–970, 1967.

Owen, C. A., Mubarak, S. J., Hargens, A. R., Rutherford, L., Garetto, L. P., and Akeson, W. H.: Intramuscular pressures with limb compression: clarification of the pathogenesis of the drug-induced muscle-compartment syndrome. N. Engl. J. Med. 300:1169–1172, 1979.

Owen, C. A., Woody, P. R., Mubarak, S. J., and Hargens, A. R.: Gluteal compartment syndromes: a report of three cases and management utilizing the wick catheter. Clin. Orthop. 132:57–60, 1978.

Penn, A. S., Rowland, L. P., and Fraser, D. W.: Drugs, coma and myoglobinuria. Arch. Neurol. 26:336–343, 1972.

Richter, R. W., Challenor, Y. B., Pearson, J., Kagen, L. J., Hamilton, L. L., and Ramsey, W. H.: Acute myoglobinuria associated with heroin addiction. J.A.M.A. 216:1172–1176, 1971.

Rowland, L. P., and Penn, A. S.: Myoglobinuria. Med. Clin. North Am. 56:1233–1256, 1972.

Schreiber, S. N., Liebowitz, M. R., and Bernstein, L. L.: Limb compression and renal impairment (crush syndrome) complicating narcotic overdose. J. Bone Joint Surg. 54-A:1683–1692, 1972.

Schreiber, S. N., Liebowitz, M. R., Bernstein, L. H., and Srinivasan, K.: Limb compression and renal impairment complicating narcotic overdose. N. Engl. J. Med. 284:368–369, 1971.

Schrier, R. W.: Principal discussant in nephrology forum: acute renal failure. Kidney Int. 15:205–216, 1979.

Weeks, S.: The crush syndrome. Surg. Gynecol. Obstet. 127:369–376, 1968.

Weiting, J.: Ueber Wundliegen Druckenkrose und Entlastung. Munch. Med Wochenschr. 65:311, 1918.

Chapter Twelve

VOLKMANN'S CONTRACTURE OF THE UPPER EXTREMITY: PATHOLOGY AND RECONSTRUCTION

Richard Gelberman, M.D.

INTRODUCTION

Volkmann's ischemic contracture of the upper extremity results from an irreversible necrosis of muscle tissue, and subsequent fibroblastic proliferation within the muscle infarct. A variable amount of longitudinal and horizontal contraction of the resulting fibrotic mass may progress over a six- to 12-month period following the injury. The necrotic muscle adheres to surrounding structures, fixing muscle position, reducing its mobility, and producing secondary compression of other structures in the region. Primary limitation of muscle excursion may lead to ultimate fixation of joint motion in a markedly limited and abnormal range.

THE CONTRACTURE

Ischemic necrosis of forearm muscles is most marked in the deep flexor compartment (Figs. 12–1, 12–2). The flexor digitorum profundus is the single most commonly and severely affected muscle. In the mildest contractures a portion of the flexor digitorum profundus may become contracted, usually involving the ring, or long and ring, fingers. In more severe contractures the long, ring, and little fingers or

The Muscles Affected in Sixteen Cases

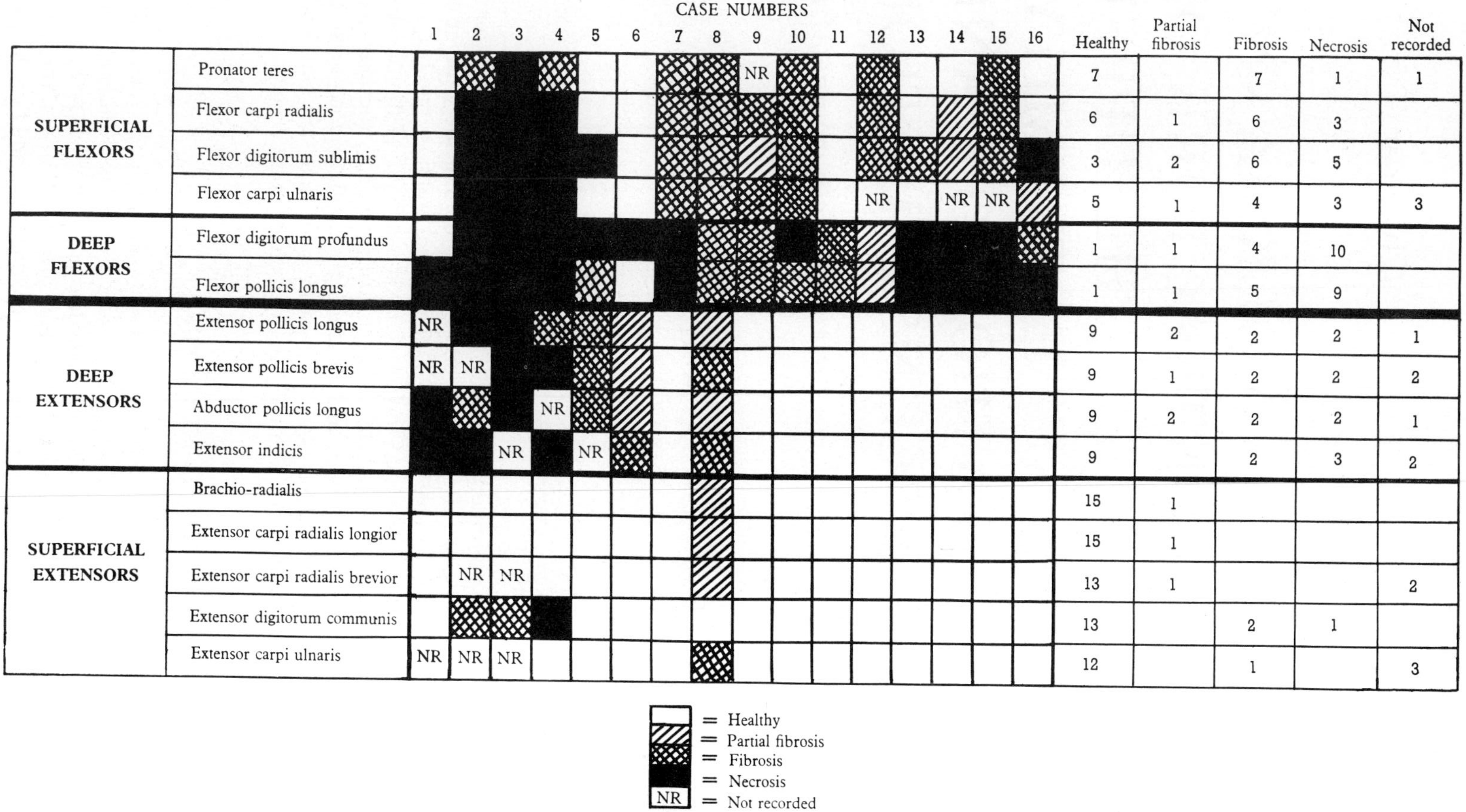

CASE NUMBERS 1–16

	Muscle	Healthy	Partial fibrosis	Fibrosis	Necrosis	Not recorded
SUPERFICIAL FLEXORS	Pronator teres	7		7	1	1
	Flexor carpi radialis	6	1	6	3	
	Flexor digitorum sublimis	3	2	6	5	
	Flexor carpi ulnaris	5	1	4	3	3
DEEP FLEXORS	Flexor digitorum profundus	1	1	4	10	
	Flexor pollicis longus	1	1	5	9	
DEEP EXTENSORS	Extensor pollicis longus	9	2	2	2	1
	Extensor pollicis brevis	9	1	2	2	2
	Abductor pollicis longus	9	2	2	2	1
	Extensor indicis	9		2	3	2
SUPERFICIAL EXTENSORS	Brachio-radialis	15	1			
	Extensor carpi radialis longior	15	1			
	Extensor carpi radialis brevior	13	1			2
	Extensor digitorum communis	13		2	1	
	Extensor carpi ulnaris	12		2	1	3

Legend:
- = Healthy
- = Partial fibrosis
- = Fibrosis
- = Necrosis
- NR = Not recorded

Figure 12–1 The muscles affected in 16 cases of Volkmann's contracture of the forearm. (With permission from Seddon, H. J.: Volkmann's contracture: treatment by incision of the infarct. J. Bone Joint Surg. 38-B:152, 1956.)

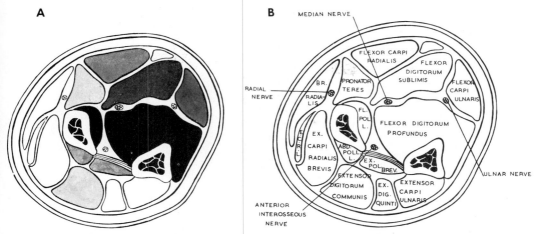

Figure 12–2   Cross-section of Volkmann's contracture of the forearm. (With permission from Seddon, H. J.: Volkmann's contracture: treatment by incision of the infarct. J. Bone Joint Surg. 38-B:152, 1956.) *A,* The shading represents the degree of involvement of the various muscles. This diagram is based on the data given in Figure 12–1 from Seddon's work. *B,* Key to muscles: the plane of section being in the upper third of the forearm.

all four digits are contracted. The flexor pollicis longus is the next most frequently involved muscle. The flexor digitorum superficialis and pronator teres generally are less severely injured. In the most generalized and severe cases of Volkmann's contracture, the wrist flexors and wrist and digital extensors may also undergo varying degrees of fibrosis and contracture.

As the swelling from the inciting compartment syndrome resolves and the affected muscles become fibrotic, the characteristic deformity of Volkmann's ischemic contracture becomes apparent. The posture of the most severely involved upper extremities consists of elbow flexion, forearm pronation, and wrist flexion (Fig. 12–3). The hand deformity consists of thumb flexion and adduction, finger metacarpophalangeal joint extension, and interphalangeal joint flexion, giving the Volkmann's clawhand appearance (Fig. 12–4).

The pathomechanics of the hand deformity in Volkmann's contracture are complex. The apparent similarity of Volkmann's and interosseous contractures has been described, but the deformities they cause are totally different. Interosseous contracture causes an intrinsic plus position, whereas Volkmann's leads to clawing of the fingers. When the two entities are associated, the resultant deformity is determined by the more powerful muscles, which are the long flexors in the case of Volkmann's contracture. Smith (1975) has described the paradoxic situation of an intrinsic plus hand with a claw deformity. The intrinsic contracture may not manifest itself until after the long flexors have been released by a muscle slide, tendon lengthening, or tenotomy. Only then will the intrinsic tightness test become positive and active interphalangeal joint flexion become difficult (Fig. 12–5).

TREATMENT OF MILD CONTRACTURES

The treatment of contractures is dependent on the severity of deformity and the time elapsed since injury. Mild deformities in which hand sensibility and strength are

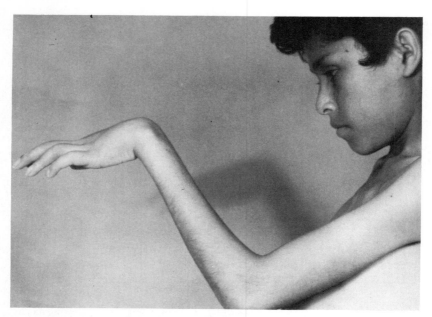

Figure 12–3 An eight year old boy with a Volkmann's ischemic contracture of the forearm, demonstrating the typical posture. This child has hemophilia, and the problem resulted from an untreated forearm hemorrhage.

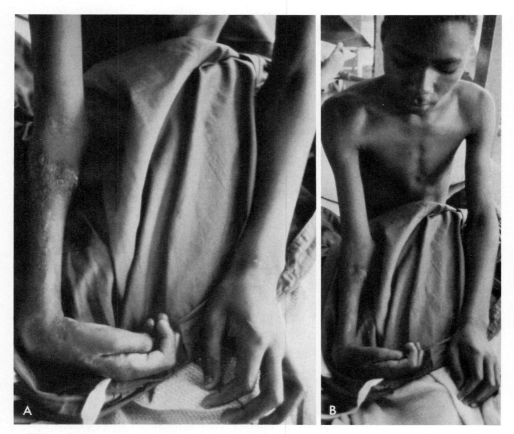

Figure 12–4 *A,* and *B,* Another patient with a Volkmann's contracture, demonstrating the deformities of the forearm and hand. (With permission from Hennessy, M., San Diego, Ca.)

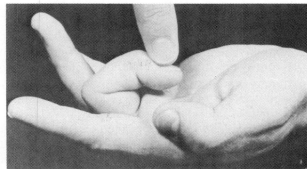

A

Figure 12–5 Test for intrinsic tightness. *A*, The first stage of the test applies passive flexion to all three joints to exclude extrinsic extensor tendon tightness. *B*, The second stage tenses the intrinsic muscles by holding the metacarpophalangeal joint in extension while applying dorsal pressure to the tip of the finger. (With permission from Flat, A. E.: The Care of the Rheumatoid Hand, 3rd ed. C. V. Mosby Co., St. Louis, 1974.)

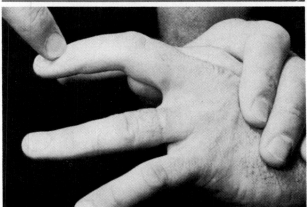

B

normal, but the deep forearm flexors are contracted, should be managed conservatively. A program of occupational therapy should include passive and dynamic extension splinting and functional training. The optimal splinting techniques for Volkmann's contracture are detailed by Goldner (1975). The goal of splinting is to maintain the wrist and interphalangeal joints in extension, increase the width of the thumb web, and provide resistance for weakened thumb intrinsics. To accomplish this, bivalved, pancake plaster casts should be alternated with low-profile digital extension and thumb opposition splints. A C-bar for maintenance of thumb position is incorporated into the plaster splint. In the early stages the patient should alternate the passive and dynamic devices in two-hour intervals during the day. He should sleep in the plaster extension splint.

Tsuge (1975) has described one indication for operative treatment in patients with mild deformities. When the contracture is limited to one or two digits, he feels that excision of the limited infarct may be helpful.

TREATMENT OF MODERATE-TO-SEVERE VOLKMANN'S CONTRACTURE WITH EVIDENCE OF NERVE COMPRESSION

The treatment of moderate-to-severe Volkmann's contracture may be divided into four phases.

Phase I: Release of Nerve Compression

In the earliest stages of treatment, attention is directed toward secondary compressive neuropathies from the infarct. Next to the extremity's vascular supply, the return of median nerve function is most closely related to the prognosis for useful extremity function. Neurologic return is related to the severity and duration of compression of neural tissue. Nerve may sustain compression for longer periods than muscle and still show some reversibility. Experience with releasing nerves before the actual treatment of the contracture has shown that nerves are capable of considerable recovery if prompt, early decompression is done (Seddon, 1956, 1973; Boyes, 1970). If the nerves are in continuity, recovery can be expected for as long as a year, and for longer periods in young patients (Seddon, 1956). Constriction of all three major forearm nerves may occur if the fibrosis is generalized and severe. A careful assessment of radial, ulnar, and median nerve function is thus essential to the first phase of treatment.

The median nerve that lies in the center of the constricting cicatrix is the most frequently and severely involved nerve in Volkmann's ischemic contracture. Compression occurs at specific locations as it passes under ligaments, through fibrous arcades, or through contracted muscles. There are four major anatomic areas that may need release in the forearm. The skin incision is the same as that used for decompression of the acute forearm compartment syndrome (see Chapter 9).

Lacertus Fibrosus. Compression at the elbow by the lacertus fibrosus is common in the acute stages of the forearm compartment syndrome, but may also occur in the later stages of contracture. The lacertus fibrosus should be decompressed if there are signs of median nerve compression.

Pronator Teres. The incidence of the median nerve passing between the humeral and ulnar heads of the pronator teres is 95 per cent. The nerve should be released completely throughout the entire length of its passage through the pronator.

Flexor Digitorum Superficialis. The median nerve is most frequently compressed beneath the fibrous origin of the flexor digitorum superficialis muscle. Peacock et al. (1969) stress the importance of the anatomic relation of the median nerve to the flexor digitorum superficialis. Because the nerve lies just beneath and within the fascia of the flexor digitorum superficialis, it may not be totally decompressed by incising investing fascia or by dissecting the flexor digitorum superficialis away from the underlying flexor digitorum profundus. Peacock et al. (1969) recommend complete nerve release and subcutaneous transplantation throughout the forearm.

Carpal Tunnel. Despite the more proximal location of most of the muscle necrosis in Volkmann's contracture, the incidence of the carpal tunnel syndrome is high. The transverse carpal ligament is incised to the midpalm as a part of the primary procedure.

Nerve stimulation is also a helpful adjunct to forearm nerve decompression. A tourniquet may be used except in the early weeks following injury (Goldner, 1975).

The incidence of ulnar and radial nerve compression is much lower than that of median nerve compression. If there are signs of ulnar motor or sensory loss, the ulnar nerve should be decompressed at the elbow as it passes between the two heads of the flexor carpi ulnaris. The radial nerve is less frequently involved, but may need decompression at the arcade of Frohse or within the supinator muscle.

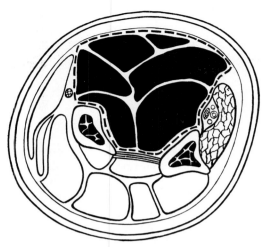

Figure 12–6 Excision of an infarct in the forearm, with preservation of the flexor carpi ulnaris and ulnar neurovascular bundle. (Reproduced by kind permission from Rev. Orthop. 46:149, 1960.)

Release of forearm neural compression should be carried out as soon as the condition of the extremity will permit. If the nerves are in continuity, some recovery can be expected. Not only is there early return of sensibility, but also a marked decrease in pain in many incidences (Goldner, 1975). If the nerve is irreparably damaged, a segment may be excised and repaired by end-to-end suture or nerve grafting.

Phase II: Treatment of Contracture

Without sensibility, increased extension through extensive release is a relatively small contribution to useful function. At the time of, or subsequent to, nerve release, attention is directed toward the release of forearm contractures. The major contractures are in the direction of elbow flexion, forearm pronation, wrist flexion, digital clawing, and thumb adduction. Correction of intrinsic hand deformities will be discussed later. The most frequently utilized procedures for the correction of forearm contractures are:
1. Infarct incision.
2. Flexor tendon lengthening, tenotomy, and tendon excision.
3. Flexor-pronator slide.

INFARCT EXCISION

Resection of the fibrotic infarct is carried out at the time of, or subsequent to, nerve release and neurolysis. Seddon (1973) recommends at least six months of preliminary traction and splinting, but Littler (1977) feels that the optimal time for infarct incision is one to several months following the injury (Fig. 12–6). The entire forearm is exposed in order to resect the functionless and contracted muscle mass. All muscles reduced to solid scar are excised. The deep flexor region of the forearm is most extensively involved in what Seddon has described as a massive, "ellipsoid-shaped" infarct. The pronator teres and pronator quadratus are released, or, if fibrotic, should be excised. The forearm may be manipulated and splinted in supination, and the wrist in extension.

FLEXOR TENDON Z-LENGTHENING, TENOTOMY, AND TENDON EXCISION

Goldner (1975) advocates tendon lengthening above the wrist. He feels that infarct incision may be unnecessary, and prefers to Z-lengthen the flexor digitorum profundus, flexor digitorum superficialis, flexor pollicis longus, and pronator teres tendons for the correction of digital contractures. Digital tendon lengthening allows extension of digits to 0 degrees, with the wrist in neutral. The flexor pollicis longus is lengthened at its musculotendinous junction to allow extension of the thumb tip while the thumb metacarpal is held in extension and external rotation. If the flexor digitorum superficialis prevents the fingers from being extended, they too should be Z-lengthened at their musculotendinous junctions. Goldner (1975) recommends consideration of flexor digitorum superficialis excision when forearm fibrosis and digital contracture is most severe.

The chief criticism of flexor tendon lengthening at the wrist is the further weakening of the already weakened flexor muscles. The release of contracture is more important than the maintenance of maximal strength, however. Tendon transfers, avoided at the time of initial release, are performed at a later time for reinforcement.

FLEXOR-PRONATOR SLIDE

The forearm muscle release originally described by Page (1923) has gained increased acceptance in recent years. Eichler and Lipscomb (1967) noted a gradual preference for this procedure over carpectomy, bone shortening, tendon lengthening, and tenotomy. Comparing the results of infarct incision at the Mayo Clinic to the muscle slide, Eichler and Lipscomb found the latter procedure more effective in obtaining a stable correction. Release involves the complete surgical detachment of the origin of the flexor muscles of the forearm from the medial epicondyle, ulna, interosseous membrane, and radius. The volar wrist capsule and pronator quadratus are also released. Tendon transfers are generally carried out secondarily.

Tsuge (1975) has extensive experience with the muscle slide, with and without infarct excision, for moderate-to-severe deformities. He performs nerve releases at the same time, and tendon transfers at a later date. He reported satisfactory-to-excellent results in a large group of moderate-to-severe contractures (Fig. 12–7). Criticisms of the flexor-pronator slide procedure include:

1. Its unpredictability, a reason for its relative unpopularity in the United States (Littler, 1977).

2. The fact that the scarred, necrotic muscle is not excised.

3. The risk of a recurrence of deformity with growth (Tsuge, 1975).

4. The resultant decrease in grip strength, particularly at the distal interphalangeal joint.

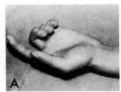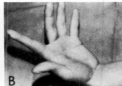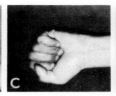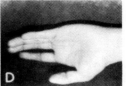

Figure 12–7 Flexion contractures of the long, ring, and little fingers after a volar forearm contusion and subsequent Volkmann's contracture. *A,* Preoperative view. *B,* When the wrist is flexed, extension of the fingers is possible. *C* and *D,* Finger flexion and extension one year after muscle-slide operation. (With permission from Tsuge, K.: Treatment of established Volkmann's contracture. J. Bone Joint Surg. 57-A:925, 1975.)

5. The possibility of incomplete correction of deformity.

Despite these drawbacks, the proponents of the flexor-pronator slide maintain that, when the procedure is done correctly, a complete and lasting correction of the wrist and digital flexion deformities of Volkmann's contracture is obtained (Page, 1923; Tsuge, 1975).

The purpose of the initial two phases of reconstruction for established ischemic contracture is to provide: (1) nerve decompression for increased sensibility, motor power, and decreased pain; (2) excision of nonviable muscle that may increase the contracture during growth; and (3) correction of flexion deformities of the wrist and fingers.

Phase III: Tendon Transfers for Substitution and Reinforcement

Tendon transfers are generally delayed until time for some nerve recovery has elapsed, and contractures have corrected by splints or release. Phalen and Miller (1947) have described a satisfactory group of transfers for digital flexion and thumb opposition. They recommend transfer of the extensor carpi radialis longus to the flexor digitorum profundus, and the extensor carpi ulnaris, prolonged by a tendon graft, to the thumb for opposition. The extensor pollicis brevis may be used to reinforce the extensor carpi ulnaris-opponens transfer. Littler (1977) advocates the restoration of opponens function by abductor digiti quinti opponens-plasty, described by Huber (1921). The extensor indicis proprius opponens-plasty described by Zancolli (1965), and later by Burkhalter (1973), is the most popular alternative.

Goldner (1975) recommends reinforcement of tendons weakened by Z-lengthening when necessary. The extensor carpi radialis longus is transferred to the flexor digitorum profundus, and the extensor carpi ulnaris is transferred to the flexor pollicis longus.

Phase IV: Salvage of Severely Contracted or Neglected Forearm

With the success of procedures in phases II and III, additional measures for the correction of severe contractures are infrequently needed. Operations that have been utilized for marked deformity are:

1. Proximal or distal row carpectomy.

2. Radius and ulna shortening.
3. Wrist fusion.
4. Digital joint fusion.

Removal of the proximal or distal rows of carpal bones may be necessary to extend the wrist to neutral while maintaining flexibility. In severe deformities, Goldner (1975) recommends removal of the carpal bones before transfer. If the extremity is too weak for transfer he advocates interphalangeal joint fusion so that the extremity can function as a hook, which is generally superior to a prosthesis.

Radius and ulna shortening and wrist fusion are no longer recommended by most authorities for the treatment of Volkmann's contracture.

RECENT ADVANCES

Free vascularized transfers of skin, nerve, and muscle have found application in Volkmann's ischemic contracture. Taylor and Daniel (1973) used a donor nerve graft with its vascular pedicle, and transferred it to the forearm with microvascular arterial and venous anastomoses. The superficial radial nerve, with its accompanying radial artery and vein, were grafted to the median nerve of a Volkmann's ischemic forearm. Significant motor and sensory return was noted.

The original report of an experimental free muscle transfer was by Tamai et al. (1970). Ch'en et al. (1977) first used the procedure for a patient with Volkmann's ischemic contracture in 1973. They transferred the lateral head of the pectoralis major to the injured forearm. Reconstruction of forearms with gracilis and rectus femoris muscles has also been described. The ultimate role for free muscle transfer, although the technique was initially promising, must await further experimentation.

RECONSTRUCTION OF HAND DEFORMITIES

After release of contractures of the long flexor tendons, the treatment of contractures within the hand are considered. The residual hand contracture may be in the form of a persistent claw deformity, with metacarpophalangeal joint extension and interphalangeal joint flexion. This is seen in the most severe deformities that are resistant to the release of forearm contractures. Frequently, the intrinsic plus deformity is encountered once the forearm is released. The etiology of the intrinsic contracture of Volkmann's ischemia is generally neurologic compression within the forearm, rather than primary intrinsic muscle necrosis in the hand (Smith, 1975). It may not be wise to release the intrinsic contracture completely, as a mild metacarpophalangeal joint deformity may prevent recurrence of the clawhand (Smith, 1975). If the intrinsic contracture is marked on clinical testing, the oblique fibers of the extensor hood are released to permit flexion of the interphalangeal joints.

Goldner (1975) recommends several procedures for the severe thumb-in-palm deformity of Volkmann's ischemic contracture. These include excision of the trapezium, metacarpophalangeal joint fusion, adductor release, and thumb web deepening. Some of the more severely affected hands should be considered for interphalangeal joint fusion.

The more significant hand disabilities are not intrinsic, but rather are secondary to forearm pathology. These include loss of median and ulnar sensibility, intrinsic paralysis secondary to ulnar and median motor paralysis, and interphalangeal joint flexion deformities secondary to long flexor contractures. Effective management of these problems, described in phases I and II, should result in significant improvements in hand function.

REFERENCES

Boyes, J. H.: Bunnell's Surgery of the Hand. J. B. Lippincott Co., Philadelphia, 1970.

Burkhalter, W. E., et al.: The extensor indicis proprius opponensplasty. J. Bone Joint Surg. 55-A:725, 1973.

Ch'en, C. W., Daniel, R. K., and Terzis, J. K.: Reconstructive Microsurgery. Little, Brown & Co., Boston, 1977.

Eichler, G. R., and Lipscomb, P. R.: The changing treatment of Volkmann's ischemic contractures from 1955 to 1965 at the Mayo Clinic. Clin. Orthop. 50:215–223, 1967.

Goldner, J. L.: *In* Flynn, J. E. (ed.): Hand Surgery. Williams & Wilkins Co., Baltimore, 1975.

Huber, E.: Hiltsoperation bei Medianers-lahmung. Dtsch. Z. Chir. 162:271, 1921.

Lister, G.: The Hand: Diagnosis and Indications. Churchill Livingstone, Edinburgh, 1977.

Littler, J. W.: The hand and upper extremity. *In* Converse, J. M. (ed.): Reconstructive Plastic Surgery. W. B. Saunders Co., Philadelphia, 1977.

Page, C. M.: An operation for the relief of flexion-contracture in the forearm. J. Bone Joint Surg. 5:233, 1923.

Peacock, E. E., Jr., Madden, J. W., and Trier, W. C.: Transfer of median and ulnar nerves during early treatment of forearm ischemia. Ann. Surg. 169:748–756, 1969.

Phalen, G. S., and Miller, R. C.: The transfer of wrist and extensor muscles to restore or reinforce flexion power of the fingers and opposition of the thumb. J. Bone Joint Surg. 29:993, 1947.

Seddon, H. J.: Volkmann's contracture: treatment by incision of the infarct. J. Bone Joint Surg. 38-B:152, 1956.

Seddon, H. J.: Surgical Disorders of the Peripheral Nerves. Williams & Wilkins Co., Baltimore, 1973.

Smith, R. J.: Intrinsic muscles of the fingers: function, dysfunction, and surgical reconstruction. Am. Acad. Ortho. Surg., Instructional Course Lectures, V. 24, 1975.

Tamai, S., Komatsu, S., Sakamoto, H., Sano, S., Sasaucki, N., Harii, Y., Tatsumi, Y., and Okuda, H.: Free muscle transplants in dogs with microsurgical, neurovascular anastamoses. Plast. Reconstr. Surg. 46:219, 1970.

Taylor, G. I., and Daniel, R. K.: The free flap: composite tissue transfer by vascular anastamoses. Aust. N. Z. J. Surg. 43:1, 1973.

Tsuge, K.: Treatment of established Volkmann's contracture. J. Bone Joint Surg. 57-A:925, 1975.

Zancolli, E.: Tendon transfers after ischemic contracture of the forearm. Classification in relation to intrinsic muscle disorders. Am. J. Surg. 109:356, 1965.

Chapter Thirteen

VOLKMANN'S CONTRACTURE OF THE LOWER EXTREMITY: PATHOLOGY AND RECONSTRUCTION

David H. Gershuni, M.D., F.R.C.S. (Eng. & Edin.)

INTRODUCTION

Richard von Volkmann's main work on ischemic muscular paralyses and contractures, published in 1881, described the condition in the upper and lower limbs. However, his first report on ischemic muscle contracture was published in 1872 and described the condition in the leg. Following deprivation of circulation to the muscle groups, the contracture was likened to postmortem stiffening. Volkmann noted that paralysis and contracture, subsequent to acute circulatory embarrassment, always appear simultaneously or follow each other closely, in contradistinction to the paralysis following nerve interruption, in which the contracture develops gradually and often very late. In the latter case the contracture provokes a deformity that can be overcome by manipulation until very late in the course. Volkmann's analogy between the stiffening of the muscles in ischemic contracture and rigor mortis is most apt, for here there is tremendous resistance to correction of the deformity from the beginning. He noted that there was some possibility for regeneration of the muscles, but that this was very slight and the tendency for fibrous replacement of the muscle and further shrinkage was much greater.

The prognosis of ischemic muscle contracture was noted by Volkmann to depend on the extent of the muscle necrosis. He felt that the final prognosis was better in the lower extremity because muscular shortening could be treated by tenotomy. Milder cases could be improved by energetic and consistent physical treatment. He suggested that new cases should be treated by the application of corrective force under chloroform anesthesia. In more established cases he cautioned that this treatment would be unsuccessful: there was a great likelihood of breaking the bones and rupturing the tendons before muscles would yield, and for these cases mechanical aids were the only means of treatment. Over 100 years later, Volkmann's contracture remains a most difficult problem to manage.

INCIDENCE

The incidence of the contracture, especially in fracture patients, seems to vary according to how diligently one looks for the condition. Ellis (1958) examined 225 cases of fracture of the tibia and noted nine patients with ischemic contracture. He further reported that one third of his 21 patients with persistent ankle and foot stiffness had clinical evidence of ischemic contracture. Owen and Tsimboukis (1967) found that 10 of 100 cases examined retrospectively had ischemic contractures. Nicholl (1964) found that, of 674 patients with tibial shaft fractures treated in a closed fashion, five had contractures related to the ankle and the foot. Griffiths (1940), Thompson and Mahoney (1951), and Horwitz (1940) also reported on the incidence of ischemic contracture following fractures. Richards (1951) found the incidence of ischemia to nerves, following injury to major arteries, to be greater in the lower than in the upper limb. Seddon (1966) noted that ischemic contracture in the lower limb occurs more often in adults than in children. Thompson and Mahoney (1951) described a group of 29 cases of which nine occurred in the lower limb in children who had sustained femoral shaft fractures.

PATHOLOGIC CHANGES OF VOLKMANN'S CONTRACTURE

Muscles

Muscle is very sensitive to ischemia. Following approximately four to six hours of total obstruction to its blood supply, necrosis will ensue (Harman, 1947; Harman and Gwinn, 1948), whereas nerves recover after six to eight hours of ischemia (Lundborg, 1970). The classic picture of a massive ellipsoidal infarct with its main axis in the length of the limb, the greatest damage at the center, and slight necrosis at the periphery is not commonly found in the leg. The circumscribed mass of ischemic tissue is usually seen when the arterial blockage is more proximal, as is found with a supracondylar fracture of the humerus in the child, which may give rise to an ellipsoidal infarct in the forearm (Seddon, 1956). Major vascular injury, compartment syndromes, laceration of muscles, or a combination of these insults may produce localized ischemia and subsequent contracture (McQuillan and Nolan, 1968). Thus, the type of muscular damage will depend on the level of the lesion, the degree and duration of the ischemia, the variable vasculature of individual muscles, and the timing and nature of specific treatment to restore the circulation. In the early stages following ischemia there is gross swelling of the muscle, which is maximal within two to four hours following the ischemia (Dahlback and Rais, 1966). The necrotic muscle is gradually replaced by scar tissues. The fibrotic infiltration occurs from the periphery of the infarct inward (Griffiths, 1940), with the muscle finishing up as a fibrous band. As occurs in many necrotic tissues, late calcification

(Horwitz, 1940; Seddon, 1964) or cyst formation within the muscle (Albert and Mitchell, 1943; Gallie and Thomson, 1960) may result.

The involvement of a particular muscle is related to its intramuscular vascular pattern. Bowden and Gutmann (1949) pointed out that the peroneal muscle group, for example, is very well supplied with blood vessels and is not often affected by ischemic contracture. Karlström et al. (1975) noted that the flexor digitorum longus and tibialis posterior were more often affected than the flexor hallucis longus. In contrast, Seddon (1966) noted that, in 15 legs affected by ischemic contracture, the flexor hallucis longus was the most often involved (60 per cent); the gastrocnemius was involved in only 20 per cent; the soleus in 25 per cent; and the other flexors, extensors, and peronei in approximately 40 per cent.

There appears to be some potential for regeneration of muscle fibers as described by Clark (1946), Hughes (1948), Bowden and Gutmann (1949), Horn and Sevitt (1951), and Sanderson et al. (1975). This regeneration depends to some extent on intramuscular anastomoses, and is severely curtailed by the coincidental production of fibrous scar tissue. Some degree of recovery begins at five to 12 days (Sanderson et al., 1975), and may be discerned clinically over a two- to six-month period following the vascular catastrophe. At this stage there will be found a graduation from total fibrous replacement of muscle to partial recovery with diffuse fibrosis and contracture, and then to nearly normal muscle. It appears that regeneration is not dependent on the muscle being innervated (Saunders and Sissons, 1953), although later workers state that muscle fibers that fail to obtain a nerve supply remain at the myotubule stage of regeneration and atrophy (Sanderson et al., 1975).

Tendons

An extensive infarct may cause necrosis of tendons, but the coincidental damage to the limb would be so severe that this tendon necrosis of itself has no significance. The fibrotic replacement of ischemic muscle may also extend to surrounding tendons and their contiguous structures (Seddon, 1964). This possibility must be taken into account in relieving contractures, by excision of tendons together with associated fibrotic muscle. Also, the fibrosis will probably interfere with any attempt at tendon transplantation.

Nerves

Meyerding (1930) considered that the nerve injury in Volkmann's ischemic contracture was due to secondary contracture of the muscle or scar compression of the nerve. However, later writers strongly disputed this, and related the neurologic deficit to preceding ischemia (Tavernier et al., 1936; Holmes et al., 1944; Seddon, 1964, 1966) and raised intracompartmental pressures (Mubarak et al., 1978). This fact, however, does not negate the possibility of coincidental traction injury to nerves following, for example, dislocation of the knee, or the possibility of laceration of a nerve from the original injury or from bone spicules and fragments. In Volkmann's contracture there is extensive and sometimes complete replacement of the Schwann tubes by collagen, which does not occur in a nerve damaged exclusively by compression (Seddon, 1964). There is some evidence that larger nerve trunks are most susceptible to ischemia (Richards, 1951; Hargens et al., 1979), as are the larger motor neurons within the nerve. In compartment syndromes, in which nerve ischemia is the result of pressure beneath the deep fascia, nerves that lie outside this fascia (e.g., the saphenous nerve) may escape damage (Kikuchi, 1978). Following severe ischemia, the nerve is shrunken and narrowed to a greater degree in the center of the infarct. The vulnerability of peripheral nerves to ischemia is considerable, and the potential for recovery of ischemic nerves is severely limited, although sensory recovery is better than motor recovery (Kikuchi, 1978). Thus, in the syndrome of Volkmann's ischemic contracture, not only is there failure of significant recovery of necrotic muscle, but also atrophy of muscles that are supplied by ischemic nerves.

Bones and Joints

Ischemia involving bone was noted by Nario (1938) when he experimentally obstructed the arterial supply of the leg in dogs. Its principal significance in the context of limb trauma is the resultant delayed healing and non-union in associated limb fractures. In children affected by Volkmann's contracture, ischemia of the physeal cartilage may diminish bone growth to the extent that a limb length discrepancy results.

There is no specific evidence that Volkmann's ischemic contracture affects the joints primarily. Akeson et al. (1958), however, showed that denervation of a limb and subsequent functional impairment give rise to atrophy and changes in the constituents of articular cartilage. Stiffness or deformity of the joints is caused by contracture of the related muscles, and limitations that the contracted muscles impose upon the joints. In some cases the reduced mobility and deformity at the joints is probably explained by minor subluxations following contracture. Thus, Karlström et al. (1975) demonstrated that this may occur at the midtarsal and subtalar joints. Walking on an equinus deformity of the foot can also give rise to hyperextension at the ipsilateral knee joint.

Vessels

Karlström et al. (1975) performed bilateral arteriography in 12 patients with Volkmann's ischemic contracture. In eight there were findings that could possibly indicate primary vascular damage. However, the arteriograms were difficult to interpret. Karlström and associates thought that minute occlusive changes in muscular branches were due to external pressure on the vessels following swelling and edema within the muscle compartments. Horn (1945) described a case of chronic ischemia of the anterior tibial muscle in a soldier who subsequently developed an acute compartment syndrome, resulting in entire necrosis of the anterior tibial and extensor hallucis longus muscles. Microscopy of the vessels in the compartment showed fibrosis of the media, adventitia, and periarterial tissues of the anterior tibial artery. The adjoining vein was also involved in a chronic inflammatory condition. Griffiths (1940) explored the vessels of four patients with established Volkmann's contracture in the forearm. In two cases the brachial artery was thrombosed. In one the internal elastic lamina was ruptured, and in the last case the artery was of normal caliber and pulsated well, although it was buried in dense scar tissue.

Skin and Nails

When affected by Volkmann's ischemic contracture, the leg may show changes of atrophy in the nails and skin. Skin ulceration may ensue from inadequate nutrition (Miller et al., 1952). Subcutaneous fat may also be replaced by scar tissue (Seddon, 1964).

CLINICAL PRESENTATION

Seddon (1966) noted that, in six of 15 cases of ischemic contracture in the leg, pain was a dominant feature, unlike the rarity of its appearance in the upper limb. The pain may be deep-seated, constant, and burning, felt only on contact between the leg and an object, or felt only on weight-bearing (Kikuchi et al., 1978). In other cases, anesthesia of the limb may be the chief complaint. Ulceration of the skin from neurotrophic or ischemic causes may also be present. A diminution in working capacity and difficulty in walking may be related to deformity and stiffness in the foot and ankle. The deformities are related to the muscle affected, the severity of the initial ischemia, and whether physical therapy or the use of an orthosis has been successful. Although the individual picture of the deformity will vary from case to case as indicated, the deformity can be described as related to the involved compartments.

Deep Posterior Compartment

The clinical picture resulting from involvement of only the long flexors of the great and other toes is one of simple toe clawing (Fig. 13–1). However, a more severe ischemic insult may produce contracture of all the muscles of the deep posterior

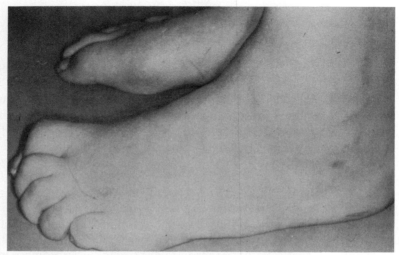

Figure 13–1   Thirteen year old boy whose original injury was a fracture of the femur complicated by a deep posterior compartment syndrome. He developed clawing of all the toes related to contractures of the long flexors.

compartment, typically giving rise to a fixed cavus, which does not disappear on standing, and a foot that is apparently shortened (Karlström et al., 1975; Matsen, 1975; Kikuchi et al., 1978). Related to this is clawing of the toes, dorsiflexion of the talus, equinus and adduction of the forefoot, and a tendency to varus of the heel (Fig. 13–2). Apparent dorsiflexion of the ankle joint is restricted because of the already dorsiflexed talus. Limited mobility of the subtalar and midtarsal joints also occurs, with fixation in an equinus attitude. The cavus of the foot is explained by the contracture of the three deep posterior compartment muscles that normally provide the main longitudinal arch support. The longitudinal arch of the foot rises, owing to the dorsiflexion of the calcaneus and the talus and increased plantar flexion occurring in the midtarsal joints, and thus makes the foot appear to shorten (Fig. 13–3). This shortens the distance between the posterior margin of the lateral malleolus and the skin over the Achilles tendon (Karlström et al., 1975). The contracture of the tibialis posterior will also cause forefoot adduction, and tend to produce medial subluxation of the tarsal joints. The contracture of the long toe flexor muscles produces the toe clawing. The maximal dorsiflexion of the talus and calcaneus together with the equinus of the forefoot, associated with subluxation of the subtalar and midtarsal

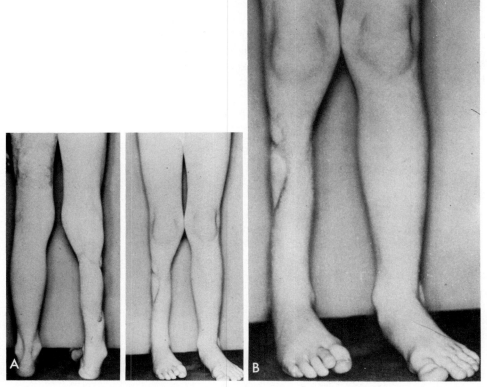

Figure 13–2 *A,* Frontal and posterior views of the legs of a 14 year old girl who ten years previously had sustained a fracture of the right femur. She had been treated in Bryant's traction, and developed a deep posterior compartment syndrome and a skin lesion that required grafting. Note the cavus of the foot, equinus, and adduction of the forefoot and varus of the hindfoot. *B,* Close-up of frontal view of the lower legs of the same girl.

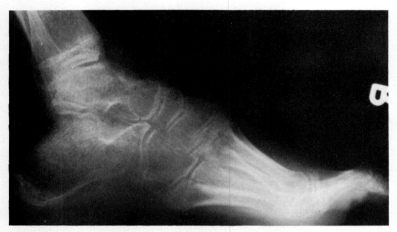

Figure 13–3   Roentgenogram of the foot of a 13 year old boy who had previously suffered from a deep posterior compartment syndrome. Note the dorsiflexion of the hindfoot and plantar flexion occurring at the midtarsal joints, producing a shortened, cavus foot. There also is accompanying clawing of the toes.

joints, explains the stiffness and limitation of motion in the foot. According to Karlström et al. (1975), when there is marked adduction deformity of the midtarsal joint, the patient voluntarily rotates the leg laterally to compensate for the adduction deformity of the foot. Seddon (1966) found that the flexor hallucis longus was the main posterior compartment muscle affected, whereas Karlström et al. (1975) found that the flexor digitorum longus and tibialis posterior were the most commonly affected; hence, the different emphasis placed on the deformities by these authors. The nerve of the deep posterior compartment is the posterior tibial nerve, and sensory changes related to this nerve damage are reflected by changes in sensation on the medial aspect of the heel, sole of the foot, and plantar aspect of the toes.

Anterior Compartment

Necrosis of the muscles of the anterior compartment will initially give rise to a footdrop. However, in the course of time as a contracture develops in this muscle group, the tendency for footdrop will decrease, and in fact contracture of the tibialis anterior will limit plantar flexion of the ankle so that splintage may be terminated. Figure 13–4 shows contracture of only the extensor hallucis longus following an anterior compartment syndrome. The deep peroneal nerve courses through the anterior compartment, and damage to its sensory component will be reflected by sensory changes in the first toe cleft.

Lateral Compartment

Although the lateral (peroneal) compartment is often affected by ischemic necrosis, no isolated deformity seems to result (Seddon, 1966). Damage to the sensory fibers in the superficial peroneal nerve, which is the main nerve of the peroneal compartment, is detected by changes in sensation of the medial side of the great toe; the second, third, and fourth toe clefts; and the dorsum of the foot. Sensation may also be altered in the territory of the deep peroneal nerve.

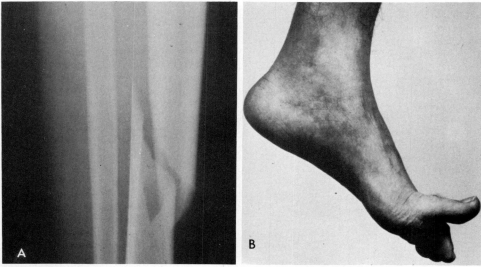

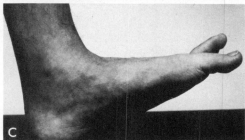

Figure 13–4 *A*, Anteroposterior roentgenogram of a closed tibial shaft fracture in a 13 year old boy. This was treated with plaster cast immobilization. *B*, Medial view of the foot one year following apparently uneventful healing of the tibial fracture. Active plantar flexion of the foot and toes leaves the great toe extended. *C*, Medial view of the foot one year following the tibial fracture, this time with foot and toes actively dorsiflexed. The great toe does not extend. The patient had sustained an anterior compartment syndrome, and subsequent ischemic contracture of the extensor hallucis longus.

Superficial Posterior Compartment

The muscles of the superficial posterior compartment are the least often affected by ischemic necrosis. However, contracture of the soleus and gastrocnemius will subsequently cause an equinovarus deformity, since the tendo Achillis insertion lies posterior and medial to the axis of the ankle joint (Fig. 13–5). When both the deep and superficial posterior compartment muscles are involved, the clinical findings are more severe, combining the features of hindfoot equinovarus with those of cavus, equinus, and adduction of the foot with toe clawing (Fig. 13–6). Weight-bearing on a persistent equinus deformity may cause hyperextension of the knee joint. Sensory changes on the lateral side of the foot reflect damage to the sural nerve, the nerve of the superficial posterior compartment.

Anesthesia and anhydrosis consistent with total or partial nerve involvement in a particular compartment will usually be found on examination. The sensory loss, however, may be present in a stocking distribution and may not always follow the distribution of the nerve associated with the particular compartment involved.

DIFFERENTIAL DIAGNOSIS

The clinical picture of an established ischemic contracture of the leg is easily diagnosed. However, milder cases may be attributed to stiffness and deformity

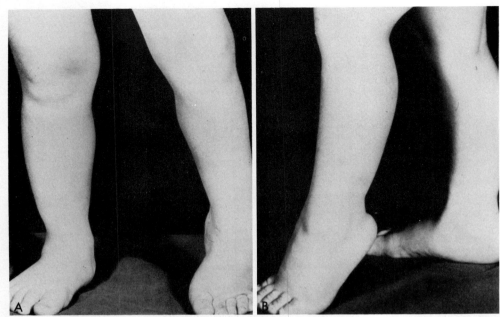

Figure 13–5 *A*, and *B*, Frontal and lateral views of a three year old child. While under treatment for meningitis he received intravenous therapy via a catheter in the left leg, which caused the development of a superficial-posterior compartment syndrome. The subsequent contracture has produced an equinovarus deformity of the left foot and ankle.

resulting from cast immobilization. We believe that many cases of partial muscle necrosis due to ischemia are not diagnosed in one or more compartments, subsequent to lower extremity fractures. Several papers discuss the chronic sequelae to tibial fractures (Seddon, 1966; Davie, 1973; Clawson, 1974; Matsen and Clawsen, 1975). Owen and Tsimboukis (1967) describe a 10 per cent incidence of ischemic muscle problems following tibial fractures in a series of 100 cases.

The sequelae of severe open injury with muscle and nerve lacerations may resemble a Volkmann's contracture. Thus, muscle contractures due to scarring following wound infection may produce a picture similar to Volkmann's contracture.

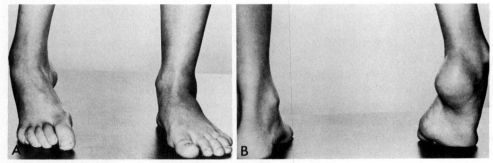

Figure 13–6 *A* and *B*, Anterior and posterior views of the right foot of a five year old girl. She originally sustained a fracture of the right femur that was complicated by deep and superficial posterior compartment syndromes. The subsequent contractures of all the posterior leg muscles have produced marked deformity consisting of hindfoot equinovarus, equinus and adduction of the forefoot, with clawing of the toes.

The extent of the muscle and nerve damage must be differentiated. The picture of a pure nerve lesion of the peroneal nerve, for example, must not be mistaken for the more complicated mixed nerve and muscle lesion of Volkmann's ischemic contracture, or vice versa. The tarsal tunnel syndrome has been described following fractures around the ankle and lower tibia (Lam, 1967), and can also be mistaken for Volkmann's ischemic contracture affecting the foot. Clawing of toes following tibial fracture may be due to intrinsic muscle weakness, nerve damage, or ischemic contracture. In addition, entrapment of the toe flexor tendons in callus at the fracture site may produce a similar picture in lower third shaft fractures (Clawson, 1974). The latter syndrome may be distinguished by the ability to extend the toes when the ankle is in plantar flexion. The clawing due to entrapment may be corrected by tendolysis at the fracture site.

Finally, the possibility of associated arterial injury, aneurysms, or arteriovenous fistulae should be investigated and diagnosed. Accurate clinical examination and selection of the appropriate investigation procedure, as described below, will allow the correct diagnosis to be made and the appropriate therapy planned.

INVESTIGATIONS TO ASSESS EXTENT OF DAMAGE

Following a careful clinical examination of the leg, it may be necessary to perform certain special investigations to define further the extent of the bone, joint, vascular, muscular, and neural damage.

Muscles

It is important to know which muscles are affected, what is the extent of the damage, and which component of the clinical picture is related to neural or muscular damage. The presence or absence of muscular recovery can be monitored by electromyography, which may show normal motor activity, dropping out of motor units, or no activity at all. However, these results cannot always be related to the clinical severity of the ischemic process, as scarring and spotty necrosis of muscle make the performance and interpretation of electromyography rather difficult.

Nerves

In certain cases a definition of the site of nerve damage may be indicated. It should be noted whether the lesion is reversible or irreversible, and the recovery should be monitored. To this end, sudomotor testing, testing of nerve conduction, strength duration curves, and electromyography may be indicated.

Following these special investigations for nerve and muscle damage, definite diagnosis of the type and extent of the injury and clear prognosis may still be impossible. In these cases an exploration of the muscle and nerve will be necessary. It should then be possible to diagnose whether nerve damage is due to traction, laceration, or ischemia. The extent of muscle damage can be determined also. Biopsies of muscle and nerve can be performed at that time, together with any surgical reconstructive procedure that may be indicated.

Bones and Joints

The site of any joint or bone deformity, the presence or absence of subluxations, and the definition of bony malunion must be known prior to the institution of any conservative or surgical procedures. Therefore, adequate radiographic examination of the leg, ankle, and foot should be performed.

Vessels

In a well established case of Volkmann's ischemic contracture, the possibilities to improve the circulation to the limb are extremely limited. Therefore, extensive examination of the vascular supply to the limb is usually unwarranted. In certain cases, skin temperature testing, oscillometry, and Doppler examination may be indicated. Femoral angiography will show no obvious arterial changes or smaller vessel occlusions. An assessment of the "runoff" will give some idea of the peripheral circulation. Angiography is also indicated if an aneurysm or arteriovenous fistula is suspected.

TREATMENT

Treatment following the acute episode should be entirely conservative, as some degree of spontaneous recovery may occur within three months or more following the acute ischemic episode. During this early period the limb should be splinted to minimize contracture and subsequent deformity (Jones, 1907). The joints should be put through a range of motion several times a day, and the affected muscles should be gently stretched. Daily galvanic stimulation of the muscles may be indicated if there is a nerve lesion (Jackson, 1945). The application of this line of treatment may well be inhibited by the limitations imposed by an associated fracture of the limb.

Following the initial, minimal three-month period of observation and conservative treatment, further assessment of the patient and the affected limb should be made. Thus, in many cases in which contractures are minimal or the patient's demands for mobility are limited, no specific treatment will be indicated. In other cases, special shoes may be needed to accommodate deformities of the foot or toes. If a drop foot is present, a brace may be required for a period. Subsequent contracture of the anterior tibial muscles will often make the drop-foot brace dispensable.

As indicated above, in order to achieve greater accuracy in diagnosis and at the same time to perform any necessary excisional or reconstructive procedure, an exploration of the leg may be required. This is performed not sooner than three months and usually at least six months following injury. The exploratory operation is done in a bloodless field. A longitudinal incision is made over the compartment involved. Exploration proceeds from superficial to deep, and necrotic muscle is excised in its entirety. If the muscles are pale and fibrotic, and contract extremely feebly or not at all when their nerve is stimulated, they also should be excised. Tendon lengthening should be performed in the case of muscles that are only partially fibrotic, but which are causing deformity. Thus, lengthening of the tendo Achillis, with or without posterior capsulotomy of the ankle joint, is often indicated for equinus deformity. Tendon transfers are only occasionally necessary in the leg (Kikuchi et al., 1978).

Insofar as it has been shown that the nerves are not being strangulated by the scar tissue, there is no indication to perform neurolysis, although exploration of the nerve may be needed for diagnostic purposes, as previously indicated. There is little place for repairing nerves in a major ischemic contracture syndrome, as the results are very poor (Seddon, 1966). Arthrodesis of the ankle joint may be performed to counteract a drop-foot deformity when the patient wishes to dispense with a drop-foot brace. Plantar fasciotomy (Horwitz, 1940), or triple arthrodesis of the foot in the more severe case of cavus or cavovarus deformity, may be indicated. If tendon lengthening or tenotomy do not improve clawing of the toes, interphalangeal arthrodesis may be performed, and Keller operation on the great toe may be required for hallux flexus (Ellis, 1958). Wedge osteotomy of the tarsus, according to the method of Cole (1940), may be used for severe forefoot equinus. Karlström et al. (1975) have described a derotational, three-dimensional osteotomy of the distal part of the tibia to normalize the functional position of the foot when a marked adduction deformity is present in the forefoot.

Amputation should be reserved for intractable pain, severe ulceration or scarring, and uncorrectible deformity (Kikuchi et al., 1978). Provided that viable skin flaps are obtainable, the condition of the underlying muscles should not influence the decision on the amputation level. Seddon (1966) noted that four of 15 cases required this radical treatment. He performed amputation below the knee with an interval of at least one year following the original injury. However, in a patient who has lost all functional muscular tissue below the knee, an amputation may sometimes be avoided. Monk (1966) describes such a case, a man who was treated by excision of muscle from all the compartments of the leg, but who had intact posterior tibial vessels and nerve, as well as sensibility over the sole, with a stiff ankle held at 90 degrees. The patient could walk well without aid and drive a tractor with his "living prosthesis."

PROGNOSIS

The prognosis depends on the relative size of the masses of viable and nonviable tissue. The potential for some regeneration of muscle fibers exists, but fibrosis may block the area of regenerating fibers. The state of the nerve supply is crucial to the final result, and recovery of nerve palsy is essential for any return of power to viable muscle and for improvement in any sensory deficit.

PROPHYLAXIS

The prevention of Volkmann's ischemic contracture in the lower extremity is dependent first on knowledge of the causative factors, and second on the early detection of signs of impending tissue necrosis. Karlström et al. (1975) have pointed out that the surgical exposure for reduction and internal fixation of leg fractures will often relieve increased intracompartmental pressure. The use of suction drains in such cases, and the ease of visual inspection and examination of the limb when a plaster cast is not necessary, are described by these authors as reasons for the low incidence of ischemic contracture in patients treated in this operative fashion.

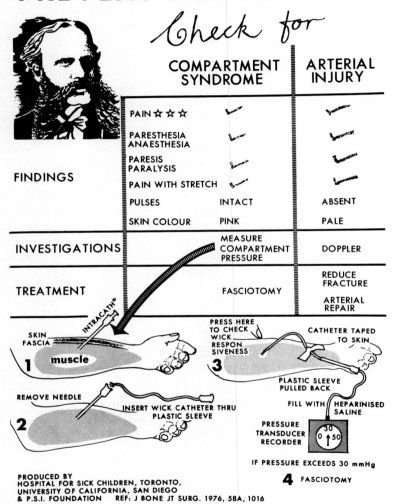

Figure 13–7 Poster outlining the clinical findings, investigations, and treatment of compartment syndromes, which is used to alert medical and nursing staff to diagnosis and prevention of Volkmann's ischemic contracture (by Rang, M., Toronto, Ont., Canada, and Mubarak, S. J., San Diego, Ca.).

Maudsley et al. (1963) have recommended the use of hyperbaric oxygen chambers for patients with severe injuries who may be susceptible to the development of ischemic necrosis of limb muscles. In the interests of earlier diagnosis and prevention of ischemic contraction, Owen and Tsimboukis (1967) have recommended that all patients with tibial shaft fractures be admitted to the hospital in the first instance, and that routine angiography should be performed during reduction of displaced tibial fractures. This latter procedure is a rather extreme and costly approach that may introduce its own additional morbidity. However, the implication that there is a greater need for early diagnosis and treatment of acute muscular ischemia can only be commended. (The indications for prophylactic fasciotomy are discussed in Chapter 10.) Above all, a high index of suspicion concerning impending ischemia, and an intimate awareness of the cardinal signs and symptoms described earlier in this book, are crucial to the prevention of Volkmann's ischemic contracture. A poster such as that of Mubarak and Rang (Fig. 13–7) should be displayed prominently on every busy accident ward as a constant reminder to housestaff, nurses, students, and attending physicians of those cardinal signs and symptoms.

REFERENCES

Akeson, W. H., Eichelberger, L., and Roma, M.: Biochemical studies of articular cartilage. II. Values following the denervation of an extremity. J. Bone Joint Surg. 40-A:153–162, 1958.

Albert, M., and Mitchell, W. R. D.: Volkmann's ischaemia of the leg. Lancet 1:519–522, 1943.

Bowden, R. E. M., and Gutmann, E.: The fate of voluntary muscle after vascular injury in man. J. Bone Joint Surg. 31-B:356–368, 1949.

Clark, W. E. L.: An experimental study of the regeneration of mammalian striped muscle. J. Anat. 80:24–40, 1946.

Clawson, D. K.: Claw toes following tibial fracture. Clin. Orthop. 103:47–48, 1974.

Cole, W. H.: The treatment of claw-foot. J. Bone Joint Surg. 22:895–908, 1940.

Dahlback, L. O., and Rais, O.: Morphologic changes in striated muscle following ischemia. Acta Chir. Scand. 131:430–440, 1966.

Davie, B. P.: Some problems in the treatment of fractures of the shaft of the tibia and fibula. Med. J. Aust. 1:997–1001, 1973.

Ellis, H.: Disabilities after tibial shaft fractures. J. Bone Joint Surg. 40-B:190–197, 1958.

Gallie, W. E., and Thomas, S.: Volkmann's ischaemic contracture: two case reports with identical late sequelae. Can. J. Surg. 3:164–166, 1960.

Griffiths, D. L. L.: Volkmann's ischaemic contracture. Br. J. Surg. 28:239–260, 1940.

Hargens, A. R., Romine, J. S., Sipe, J. C., Evans, K. L., Mubarak, S. J., and Akeson, W. H.: Peripheral nerve-conduction block by high muscle-compartment pressure. J. Bone Joint Surg. 61-A:192–200, 1979.

Harman, J. W.: A histological study of skeletal muscle in acute ischemia. Am. J. Pathol. 23:551–565, 1947.

Harman, J. W., and Gwinn, R. P.: The recovery of skeletal muscle fibers from acute ischemia as determined by histological and chemical methods. Am. J. Pathol. 25:741–755, 1948.

Holmes, W., Highet, W. B., and Seddon, H. J.: Ischaemic nerve lesions occurring in Volkmann's contracture. Br. J. Surg. 32:259–275, 1944.

Horn, C. E.: Acute ischaemia of the anterior tibial muscle and the long extensor muscles of the toes. J. Bone Joint Surg. 27-B:615–622, 1945.

Horn, J. S., and Sevitt, S.: Ischaemic necrosis and regeneration of the tibialis anterior muscle after rupture of the popliteal artery. J. Bone Joint Surg. 33-B:348–358, 1951.

Horwitz, T.: Ischemic contracture of the lower extremity. Arch. Surg. 41:945–959, 1940.

Hughes, J. R.: Ischaemic necrosis of the anterior tibial muscles due to fatigue. J. Bone Joint Surg. 30-B:581–594, 1948.

Jackson, S.: The role of galvanism in the treatment of denervated voluntary muscle in man. Brain 68:300, 1945.

Jones, R.: On a simple method of dealing with Volkmann's ischemic paralysis. Am. J. Orthop. Surg. 5:377–383, 1907.

Karlström, G., Lönnerhold, T., and Olerud, S.: Cavus deformity of the foot after fracture of the tibial shaft. J. Bone Joint Surg. 57-A:893–900, 1975.

Kikuchi, S., Hasue, M., and Watanabe, M.: Ischemic contracture in the lower limb. Clin. Orthop. 134:185–192, 1978.

Lam, S. J. S.: Tarsal tunnel syndrome. J. Bone Joint Surg. 49-B: 87–92, 1967.

Lundborg, G.: Ischemic nerve injury. Ph.D. thesis, University of Gothenburg, 1970.

Matsen, F. A.: Compartmental syndrome. A unified concept. Clin. Orthop. 113:8–14, 1975.

Matsen, F. A., III, and Clawson, D. K.: The deep posterior compartmental syndrome of the leg. J. Bone Joint Surg. 57-A:34–39, 1975.

Maudsley, R. H., Hopkinson, W. I., and Williams, K. G.: Vascular injury treated with high pressure oxygen in a mobile chamber. J. Bone Joint Surg. 45-B:346, 1963.

McQuillan, W. M., and Nolan, B.: Ischaemia complicating injury. A report of 37 cases. J. Bone Joint Surg. 50-B:482–492, 1968.

Meyerding, H. W.: Volkmann's ischemic contracture. J.A.M.A. 94:394–400, 1930.

Miller, D. S., Markin, L., and Grossman, E.: Ischemic fibrosis of the lower extremity in children. Am. J. Surg. 84:317–322, 1952.

Monk, C. J. E.: Traumatic ischaemia of the calf. J. Bone Joint Surg. 48-B:150–152, 1966.

Mubarak, S. J., Owen, C. A., Hargens, A. R., Garetto, L. P., and Akeson, W. H.: Acute compartment syndromes, diagnosis and treatment with the aid of the wick catheter. J. Bone Joint Surg. 60-A:1091–1095, 1978.

Nario, C. V.: Ann. Fac. Med. Montevideo 10:560, 1925. Reprinted in greater part in J. Int. Chir. 3:87, 1938.

Nicholl, E. A.: Fractures of the tibial shaft. A survey of 705 cases. J. Bone Joint Surg. 46-B:373–387, 1964.

Owen, R., and Tsimboukis, B.: Ischaemia complicating closed tibial and fibular shaft fractures. J. Bone Joint Surg. 49-B:268–275, 1967.

Richards, R. L.: Ischaemic lesions of peripheral nerves: a review. J. Neurol. Neurosurg. Psychiatry 14:76–87, 1951.

Sanderson, R. A., Foley, R. K., McIvor, G. W. D., and Kirkaldy-Willis, W. H.: Histological response on skeletal muscle to ischemia. Clin. Orthop. 113:27–35, 1975.

Saunders, J. H., and Sissons, H. A.: Effect on denervation on regeneration of skeletal muscle after injury. J. Bone Joint Surg. 35-B:113–124, 1953.

Saunders, J. T.: Etiology and treatment of clawfoot. Report of the results in 102 feet treated by anterior tarsal resection. Arch. Surg. 30:179–198, 1935.

Seddon, H. J.: Volkmann's contracture: treatment by excision of the infarct. J. Bone Joint Surg. 38-B: 152–174, 1956.

Seddon, H. J.: Volkmann's ischaemia. Br. Med. J. 1:1587–1592, 1964.

Seddon, H. J.: Volkmann's ischaemia in the lower limb. J. Bone Joint Surg. 48-B:627–636, 1966.

Tavernier, L., Dechaume, J., and Pouzet, F.: Infarctus musculaires et lesions nerveuses dans le syndrome de Volkmann. J. Med. Lyon 17:815, 1936.

Thompson, S. A., and Mahoney, L. J.: Volkmann's ischaemic contracture and its relationship to fracture of the femur. J. Bone Joint Surg. 33-B:336–347, 1951.

Volkmann, R. von: Die Krankenheiten der Bewegungsorgane. *In* Handbuch der Allegemeinen und Specillen Chirurgie, Pitha-Billroth 2:846, 1872.

Volkmann, R. von: Die ischaemischen Muskellähmungen und Kontrakturen. Zentralb. Chir. 8:801, 1881.

Chapter Fourteen

EXERTIONAL COMPARTMENT SYNDROMES

Scott J. Mubarak, M.D.

The exercise-initiated compartment syndromes are divided into two forms with regard to clinical findings and reversibility. An acute syndrome exists when intracompartmental pressure is elevated to a level and duration such that immediate decompression is necessary to prevent intracompartmental necrosis. The clinical findings and course are the same as a compartment syndrome initiated by a fracture or contusion, except that the condition occurs following strenuous activities, and there is no external trauma. The second form, a chronic (or recurrent) compartment syndrome, arises when exercise raises intracompartmental pressure sufficiently to produce small vessel compromise and therefore ischemia, pain, and (on rare occasions) neurologic deficit. These symptoms disappear when the activity is stopped and reappear during the next period of exercise. However, if the exercise is continued despite pain (i.e., with continued ischemia), a chronic compartment syndrome may proceed to an acute form that requires decompression. An example of the latter is the military recruit who exercises under duress beyond his own limits of pain tolerance.

HISTORY

An anterior compartment syndrome initiated by exertion was probably first described by Dr. Edward Wilson (Fig. 14–1), the medical officer on Capt. R. F. Scott's ill-fated race to the South Pole (Freedman, 1953). Scott, Wilson, and three others failed in their attempt to reach the South Pole before the Norwegian, Roald Amundsen (Fig. 14–2). On the return trip from the Pole, Dr. Wilson began experiencing severe pain and swelling in the area of the anterior compartment, which he accurately described in his diary. The following is an excerpt from his diary dated January 30, 1912:

My left leg exceedingly painful all day so I gave Birdie my ski and hobbled alongside the sledge on foot. The whole of the tibialis anticus is swollen and tight, and full of tenosynovitis, and the skin red and oedematous over the shin.

209

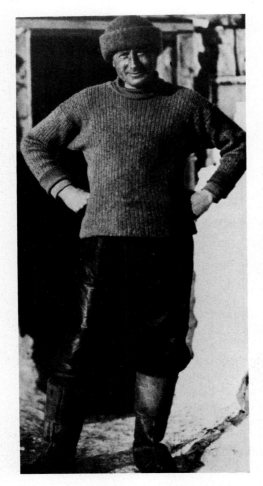

Figure 14–1 Dr. Edward Wilson unknowingly was the first to describe the effects of an anterior compartment syndrome. He was the medical officer for Capt. R. F. Scott's South Pole expedition of 1911–12. (With permission from Brent, P.: Captain Scott. Saturday Review Press, New York, 1974.)

Over the ensuing days the leg gradually became less painful as his general medical condition deteriorated. Dr. Wilson perished along with Scott and the others in the expedition on their return trip from the Pole.

Thirty years passed before the exertional anterior compartment syndrome of the leg became recognized as an entity. In a lecture, Vogt (1943) described a case of ischemic muscle necrosis following marching (Table 14–1). Horn (1945) added two more cases, one involving the anterior and lateral compartment, and an isolated case of the anterior compartment. The previous year, Sirbu et al. (1944) described a case of the anterior compartment syndrome resulting from a long march. Sirbu performed a fasciotomy and termed the disorder "march synovitis." Over the next 15 years many isolated cases of acute anterior compartment syndromes of the leg resulting from exertion were reported (Severin, 1944; Hughes, 1948; Carter et al., 1949; Tillotson and Coventry, 1950; Kornstad, 1955; Kunel and Lynn, 1958). Only two cases of the acute syndrome with lateral compartment involvement have been noted (Blandy and Fuller, 1957), along with only one case involving the superficial posterior compartment (Mubarak et al., 1978A).

Mavor (1956) probably described the first chronic form of the anterior exertional compartment syndrome. His patient had recurring pain in the anterior compartment

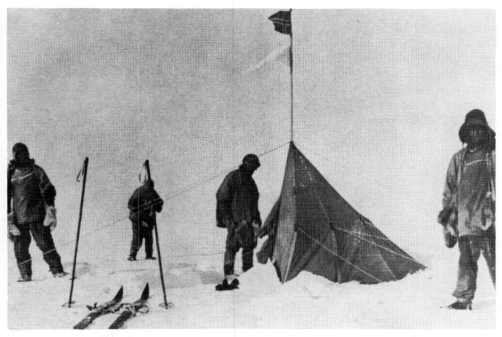

Figure 14–2 Dr. Wilson, Capt. Scott, and others view the flag and tent of their competition (the Norwegian, Amundsen) at the South Pole on Jan. 17, 1912. These explorers perished on their return trip from the Pole. Dr. Wilson was hobbled by the effects of an anterior compartment syndrome. (With permission from Brent, P.: Captain Scott. Saturday Review Press, New York, 1974.)

associated with numbness and muscle hernia. Fasciotomy relieved the problem. The existence of a chronic syndrome was questioned by Griffiths (1956) and later by Grunwald and Silberman (1959). However, subsequent reports by various authors and the pressure studies of French and Price (1962) confirmed the existence of this entity. In his monograph on this subject, Reneman (1968) reported more than 61 chronic cases also with pressure documentation.

A chronic form involving other compartments of the leg has been described, although tissue pressure documentation is lacking. Reneman (1968) reported seven

Table 14–1 HISTORICAL DESCRIPTION OF EXERTIONAL
COMPARTMENT SYNDROMES OF THE LEG

Compartment	Acute Form	Chronic Form
Anterior	Wilson (1912)* Vogt (1943) Sirbu et al. (1944) Horn (1945)	Mavor (1956)
Lateral	Blandy and Fuller (1957)	Reneman (1968)
Superficial Posterior	Mubarak et al. (1978A)	Kirby (1970)
Deep Posterior	—	—

*Freedman (1953).

cases of the chronic compartment syndrome involving both the lateral and anterior compartments. Kirby (1970) described a patient with bilateral, chronic superficial posterior compartment syndromes, whose symptoms were relieved by fasciotomies. Three additional cases of chronic syndromes in the superficial posterior compartment were reported by Snook (1975). Eleven cases of exertional syndromes involving the deep posterior tibial compartment were detailed by Puranen (1974) (see discussion of the medial tibial syndrome to follow).

Isolated chronic cases involving the second interosseous compartment of the hand (Reid and Travis, 1973) and the volar compartment of the forearm (Tompkins, 1977) have also been documented.

PATHOGENESIS

The exact pathogenesis of the exertional tibial compartment syndrome is unknown. Elevated compartmental pressure is the immediate cause of muscle and nerve ischemia in acute compartment syndromes. Furthermore, studies of patients with chronic syndromes in our laboratory (Mubarak and Hargens, 1980) and by others (French and Price, 1962; Reneman, 1975) have shown elevated pressures in the involved compartments at rest, as well as higher pressures sufficient to precipitate symptoms during and after exertion. The factors responsible for the elevation of compartmental pressure in certain individuals following exercise remain speculative. Intracompartmental pressure rises as a consequence of: (1) the limitation of the compartment size (rigid container); and (2) an increase in volume of the contents of the compartment (Table 14–2).

The rigid container in the usual case is the anterior compartment of the leg. This volume is enclosed in a noncompliant, osteofascial envelope comprising the anterior compartment fascia, the interosseous ligament, the tibia, and the fibula. There is little room for expansion, so that a small amount of fluid accumulation in this space will cause an abrupt rise in pressure.

During exercise two interesting phenomena occur. First, during a strong isometric or isotonic contraction, intracompartmental pressure rises sufficiently to render the muscle ischemic while the contraction is maintained. This conclusion has been reached by a number of authors using a variety of indirect methods of estimating tissue pressure (Anrep et al., 1934; Grant, 1938; Wells et al., 1938; Barcroft and Millen, 1939; Hill, 1948; Kjellmer, 1964; Ashton, 1975). However, we confirmed this by direct measurement of the muscle during contraction in our own laboratory, utilizing the wick catheter (Mubarak et al., 1976; Owen et al., 1981;

Table 14–2 PROBABLE FACTORS IN THE PATHOGENESIS OF
THE EXERTIONAL COMPARTMENT SYNDROME

A. Limited Compartment Size
    1. Thickened Fascia
B. Increased Volume of Compartment Contents
    1. Acutely — Muscle swelling due to increased capillary permeability
           and intracellular edema
    2. Acutely — Restricted venous or lymphatic outflow
    3. Acutely — Hemorrhage due to torn muscle fibers
    4. Chronically — Muscle hypertrophy

Schmidt et al., 1981) (Fig. 14–3). During an acute muscle contraction, intracompartmental pressure probably rises as a result of tissue compression and a cessation of blood flow out of the muscle.

Second, with prolonged exercise, muscle bulk increases by as much as 20 per cent acutely (Wright, 1961). Linge (1959) demonstrated acute hypertrophy in untrained rats after five hours of exercise. These findings probably reflect increased capillary permeability resulting in fluid accumulation in both intracellular and extracellular spaces. Other possibilities have been suggested to account for the volume increase in the compartment of subjects under exercise conditions. Anomalies of venous or lymphatic return may exist in patients with the chronic syndrome (Reneman, 1968). Unaccustomed exercise may lead to hemorrhage from torn muscle fibers as an additional source of fluid accumulation (Pearson et al., 1948; Carter et al., 1949). Finally, in the trained athlete whose muscles have hypertrophied, there is less room in the compartments to accommodate the acute swelling (Fig. 14–4). Whatever the causes, the well documented pressure increases indicate that fluid must accumulate in the compartment interstitial spaces to cause either chronic or acute compartment syndromes, or both, following exertion.

EXERTIONAL TIBIAL COMPARTMENT SYNDROME: ACUTE FORM

Excessive use of muscles as a cause of an acute compartment syndrome is uncommon. Less than 100 cases are documented in the literature, and in our study of over 80 patients with acute syndromes over the past six years, only two cases have been initiated by exercise.

Most cases of the acute syndrome in the literature developed in patients performing unaccustomed tasks (forced marches or prolonged runs). In some cases

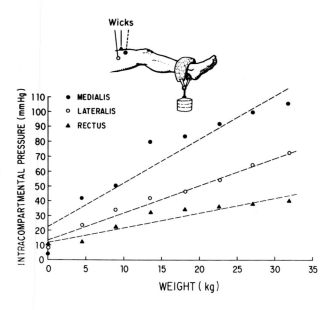

Figure 14–3 Wick catheters were inserted into three different muscles of the quadriceps. Increasing weight on the foot during straight leg-raising caused a directly proportional increase in intramuscular pressure in these muscles. With weights greater than 15 kg, the pressure in all three muscles tested exceeded capillary blood pressure (25 to 30 mm Hg). (From Schmidt, D. A., et al.: An assessment of isometric quadriceps exercises. Unpublished data, 1981.)

QUADRICEPS FEMORIS

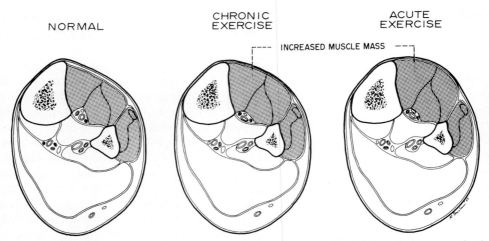

Figure 14-4 In the trained athlete whose muscles have hypertrophied there is less room in the compartments to accommodate the acute swelling that occurs during exercise.

the patient had symptoms of a chronic compartment syndrome for months before the acute episode (Reneman, 1968). The initial symptom of this acute compartment syndrome is severe pain over the involved compartment. The pain either begins during the exercise or develops within 12 hours afterward. As pain increases, numbness and weakness are noted and medical attention is sought.

The clinical findings, laboratory investigations, and treatment of the acute exertional compartment syndrome are identical to those of an acute syndrome of any cause, and have been covered in preceding chapters.

EXERTIONAL TIBIAL COMPARTMENT SYNDROME: CHRONIC FORM

Background and Clinical Presentation

The chronic or recurrent syndrome is much more common than the acute form. Reneman (1968, 1975) reported the largest series (61 cases), and nearly all involved the anterior compartment only. Symptoms were bilateral in 95 per cent of his cases, and about 75 per cent of ours. Most of Reneman's patients were from the military, whereas ours range from casual joggers to enthusiastic marathon runners. The majority are males.

In most cases the patient notes recurrent pain over the anterior or lateral compartment area that is initiated by exercise. Symptoms have usually been present for months by the time medical attention is sought. The exercise may vary from a prolonged walk or march to a marathon run. For a given patient the onset of the pain is reproducible for a specific speed and distance. Usually it is necessary for the patient to discontinue his run and rest for a few minutes. However, this set of events varies, and some individuals can continue to run at a reduced speed, whereas others who discontinue their exercise may be bothered by symptoms immediately. These symptoms may last for hours.

The pain is described as a feeling of either pressure, aching, cramping, or a stabbing sensation over the anterior compartment. Occasionally, associated symptoms include numbness on the dorsum of the foot, weakness, or an actual foot drop.

The findings on physical examination prior to exercise are few. Neurocirculatory examinations are normal. Usually the muscles are well developed in all compartments. It is best to ask the patient to perform the usual run or exercise that initiates the problem. Postexercise a sensation of increased fullness over the anterior compartment may be noted, but the neurocirculatory status usually remains normal. Occasionally, hypoesthesia on the dorsum of the foot will be documented. Changes in the pedal pulses after exercise require further work-up of the vascular system.

Muscle hernias, noted in 60 per cent of Reneman's cases (1968), may be clinically more obvious after exercise. We have encountered these fascial defects much less frequently (20 per cent) (Mubarak and Hargens, 1980). Most are located in the lower third of the leg overlying the anterior intramuscular septum between the anterior and lateral compartments (Fig. 14–5). In this location the fascial defect may represent an enlargement of the orifice through which a branch of the superficial peroneal nerve (medial dorsal cutaneous nerve) exits the lateral compartment. We have encountered this situation on three occasions. The muscle herniation may cause superficial peroneal nerve irritation and even neuroma formation (Garfin et al., 1977) (Figs. 14–6, 14–7).

Laboratory Investigations of Chronic Compartment Syndrome

Tissue Pressure Measurement.   The study of chronic syndromes by means of the needle technique was first undertaken by French and Price (1962). Reneman

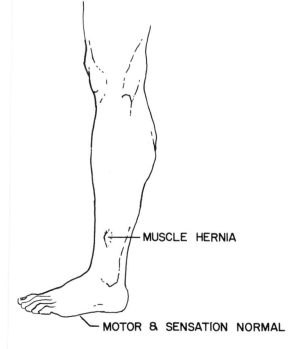

Figure 14–5 Muscle hernias are commonly associated with chronic exertional compartment syndromes. The neurologic examination is usually normal.

MUSCLE HERNIA

MOTOR & SENSATION NORMAL

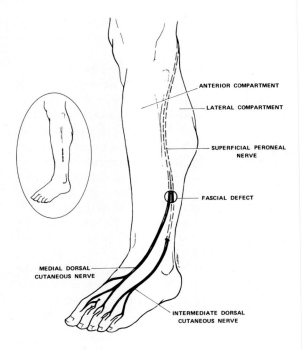

ANTERIOR COMPARTMENT

LATERAL COMPARTMENT

SUPERFICIAL PERONEAL
NERVE

FASCIAL DEFECT

MEDIAL DORSAL
CUTANEOUS NERVE

INTERMEDIATE DORSAL
CUTANEOUS NERVE

Figure 14–6 Relationship of superficial peroneal nerve branches to fascial defect, commonly seen with chronic exertional compartment syndromes. *Inset*: Incision used for fasciotomy and exploration of the defect and nerves. (From Garfin, S. R., et al.: Exertional anterolateral-compartment syndrome. J. Bone Joint Surg. 59-A:404–405, 1977.)

(1968), using the same technique, investigated a large number of patients. He found that intracompartmental pressures at rest, immediately after exercise, and at six minutes postexercise exceeded those of normal control subjects of comparable age. He could not measure the pressures continuously during exercise with this technique, however.

Utilizing the wick catheter technique (Mubarak et al., 1978B), we have observed similar changes in pressure between the two groups, with the additional advantages of continuous monitoring during the exercise. The wick catheter is inserted into the involved compartment under sterile conditions and local anesthesia. It is taped into position, and pressure measurements are determined during complete rest in the supine position. The patient's foot is then attached to an isokinetic exerciser* using

---

*Orthotron, made by Lumex Corporation.

Figure 14–7 Intraoperative photograph of fascial defect, bulging peroneus brevis, and medial dorsal cutaneous nerve exiting from the defect *(see probe, left)*. The intermediate dorsal cutaneous nerve *(right)* has developed a neuroma. (From Garfin, S. R., et al.: Exertional anterolateral-compartment syndrome. J. Bone Joint Surg. 59-A:404–405, 1977.)

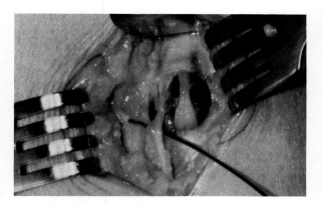

the foot attachment apparatus (Fig. 14–8). A standard setting is used for all patients. The individual is instructed to dorsiflex and plantar-flex the foot once every two seconds, until the actions are terminated by pain or fatigue. The pressures are continuously recorded by the wick catheter, which is connected to a pressure transducer and strip recorder. We have found this method of exercise the most standard, although on occasion we have employed a treadmill or had the patient run his "usual" distance to initiate the pain. Reinsertion of the wick in these circumstances must be rapid, since intracompartmental pressure falls quickly.

The mean rest pressure of the anterior compartment in the supine position of normal subjects is 4 ± 4 mm Hg. During exercise, pressure rises to more than 50 mm Hg. Moreover, intracompartmental pressure rises and falls with each muscular contracture and relaxation. Upon terminating the exercise through fatigue or pain, intracompartmental pressure begins to fall. In normal subjects the pressure will decline below 30 mm Hg immediately, and after five minutes pressure will be back to the pre-exercise rest levels in most cases (Fig. 14–9).

Resting intracompartmental pressure is usually greater than 15 mm Hg in patients with the chronic syndrome. During exercise these pressures rise above 75 mm Hg. At times during exercise they may exceed 100 mm Hg. At completion of the exercise, intracompartmental pressure will remain greater than 30 mm Hg for five minutes or longer, and symptoms of pain and possibly paresthesia are usually present (Fig. 14–9). We have used these findings as our laboratory confirmation of the chronic compartment syndrome. In these patients we recommend fasciotomy, to normalize both resting and postexercise intracompartmental pressure.

Venography. This was employed by Reneman (1968) in his study of the chronic syndrome. When neither of the anterior tibial veins filled at two or four minutes after exercise, he considered this diagnostic of a chronic syndrome (Fig. 14–10). Although an interesting investigation, the technique has flaws and is much more invasive than tissue pressure measurement.

Electromyography and Nerve Conduction. Leach et al. (1967) reported one

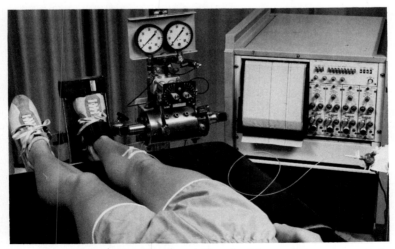

Figure 14–8 The wick catheter has been inserted into the right anterior compartment of a patient with a suspected chronic compartment syndrome. Foot is attached to an isokinetic exerciser. Intracompartmental pressures are continuously recorded by the wick catheter, connected to a pressure transducer and strip recorder located on the patient's right.

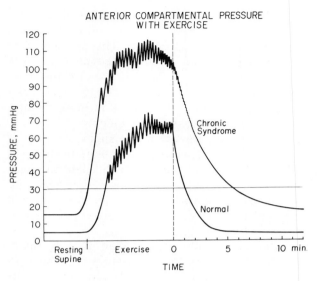

ANTERIOR COMPARTMENTAL PRESSURE
WITH EXERCISE

Figure 14–9 Illustrative anterior compartmental pressures recorded with the wick catheter during exercise of a normal subject and a patient afflicted with a chronic anterior compartment syndrome. The resting pressure of the chronic syndrome is elevated over that of the normal control. During exercise the pressure rises to greater than 75 mm Hg, and remains greater than 30 mm Hg for more than five minutes in the patient with the chronic syndrome.

patient who demonstrated denervation potentials in the anterior compartment. Reneman (1968) utilized this in five patients. He could demonstrate no abnormality either at rest or during exercise. We agree that electromyography is of little value, although nerve conduction may be helpful if there is a subjective neurologic deficit in patients with a possible chronic compartment syndrome.

Figure 14–10 Reneman performed venograms on patients with suspected chronic compartment syndromes. At rest the anterior tibial veins filled *(left)*. If, at four minutes after exercise, the anterior tibial veins are not yet filled, he considers this diagnostic of a chronic anterior compartment syndrome. (With permission from Reneman, R. S.: The Anterior and the Lateral Compartment Syndrome of the Leg. Mouton Co., The Hague, 1968.)

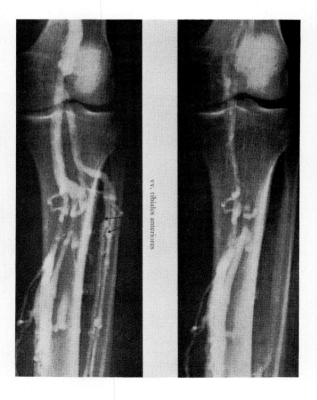

Sodium[22] Chloride Clearance. French and Price (1962) and Kennelly and Blumberg (1968) demonstrated reduced clearance of sodium[22] chloride after exercise, but no change at rest when compared to normals. We have had no experience with this technique.

Differential Diagnosis of Chronic Compartment Syndrome

Intermittent Claudication due to Partial Femoral Artery Obstruction. The history of this condition is identical except that patients tend to be a little older than chronic syndrome patients. The diagnostic clue in this entity is that the pedal pulses are present at rest, but disappear with exercise. An arteriogram will confirm this diagnosis.

Stress Fractures of the Tibia or Fibula. This diagnosis can be made clinically by noting local tenderness over the bone at the fracture site. Although the radiographs will be negative initially, changes will usually be demonstrated 10 to 14 days after onset of pain. A bone scan will generally be positive at the onset and may be beneficial in the diagnosis.

Tenosynovitis. Tenosynovitis of the dorsiflexors of the foot will be characterized by crepitus, erythema, and pain on movement of these tendons.

Infection. Cellulitis, pretibial fever (Daniels and Grennan, 1934), and tropical diseases (Browne, 1962) may suggest a compartment syndrome initially. In most cases, however, the patient will be febrile, with the loss of function secondary to pain. These conditions are rarely confused with the chronic syndrome.

Shin Splints. These are usually defined as the pain associated with activity at the beginning of the "season" after a relatively inactive period (Slocum, 1967). Pain and tenderness are generally located over the anterior compartment, and these symptoms clear in a couple of weeks as the athlete becomes conditioned. The pain is not claudicatory, i.e., it starts immediately with activity, not after running a given distance. Reneman (1968) feels that shin splints may represent a mild form of the chronic compartment syndrome, but our preliminary studies have not documented increased pressure in patients with shin splints.

Medial Tibial Syndrome. This syndrome has been classified by various authors as a stress fracture (Devas, 1958), deep posterior compartment syndrome (Puranen, 1974), or a shin splint (Slocum, 1967; Andrish et al., 1974; Jackson and Bailey, 1975). Because the etiology is unknown, the terminology selected by Puranen, "medial tibial syndrome," is probably most appropriate for this affliction.

It is usually seen in runners, but has also been noted in athletes participating in tennis, volleyball, basketball, and long-jumping. The pain is recurrent and associated with repetitive strenuous exercise. It is located along the medial border of the distal tibia. It increases after running a given distance and decreases with rest. Pain is often present even without exercise when the posteromedial edge of the distal tibia is palpated.

The physical findings are very specific. There is a localized area of tenderness over the posteromedial edge of the distal third of the tibia (Fig. 14–11). This area is frequently indurated and exquisitely tender. Atrophy of the posterior compartment muscles is sometimes noted. No motor, sensory, or circulatory disturbance is found. On examination of the patient following exertion, the painful area will be more symptomatic. Injection of Xylocaine into this area will relieve the pain and allow the patient to exercise without discomfort.

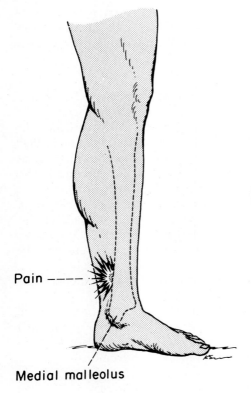

Pain ----

Medial malleolus

Figure 14–11 Clinical findings of the medial tibial syndrome. There is a localized area of tenderness over the posterior medial edge of the distal third of the tibia.

Radiographs are always normal initially. If the duration of the pain exceeds three to four weeks, hypertrophy of the cortex and some periosteal new bone formation may be noted. Devas (1958) presented a series of patients who had evidence of a stress fracture of the tibial cortex in this area. Bone scanning (Fig. 14–12) may demonstrate a mild uptake or may be entirely normal (Puranen, 1974; Mubarak and Hargens, 1980). However, even when positive, bone scan uptake is not as increased as with a stress fracture.

Tissue pressure measurement has been performed by D'Ambrosia et al. (1977) using the needle technique. In this series, rest pressures in the deep posterior compartment in 14 athletes were all within normal limits. Ericksson and Wallensten (1979) also have noted "normal" pressure studies in patients with the medial tibial syndrome. Similarly, in a series of 14 patients with this symptom complex whom we have studied, the rest and postexercise pressures have remained well within normal limits. Our mean rest pressure was 8 mm Hg, and immediately postexercise it was 9 mm Hg. During exercise, pressure rose to an average of 55 mm Hg.

Devas (1958) was one of the first to report on patients with the medial tibial syndrome. He believed that this entity represented an incomplete fracture involving one cortex of the tibia. Fourteen of his patients demonstrated radiographic changes in the lower third of the tibia medially. In nine patients he was able to demonstrate an actual fracture line, and in five others, only periosteal reaction. Jackson and Bailey (1975) agreed with Devas that this represented an atypical stress fracture. Although only one of their athletes demonstrated a fracture line, follow-up films on many others showed periosteal new bone formation and the cortical hypertrophy typical of

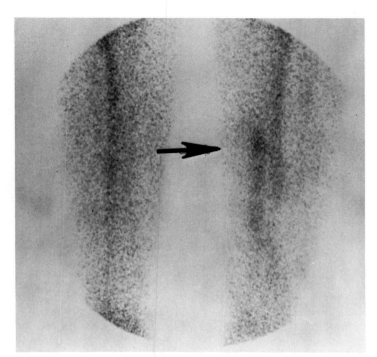

Figure 14–12 Technetium pyrophosphate bone scan from a patient with the medial tibial syndrome. There is a diffuse and mild uptake along the distal third of the medial tibia *(see arrow).*

this entity. Clement (1974) believed that this represented a periostitis, and that with continued stress or overloading, a typical stress fracture could result.

Without pressure measurement documentation, Puranen (1974) theorized that this syndrome represented a deep posterior compartment syndrome. His rationale was based primarily on the mild uptake from the strontium bone scans and negative radiographs in these patients. Puranen noted that the radiographs of typical stress fractures are more obvious than those of this syndrome. Furthermore, he had excellent results in all 11 patients in whom he had performed a deep posterior compartment fasciotomy. Since then, however, intracompartmental pressure studies of D'Ambrosia et al. (1977), Ericksson and Wallensten (1979), and our laboratories (Mubarak and Hargens, 1980) refute the possibility that this is a deep posterior compartment syndrome.

Biopsy material from two of our patients who underwent fasciotomy demonstrated inflammation and a vasculitis on microscopic examination in the area of tenderness (Fig. 14–13). This finding, the mildly positive bone scans, and the radiographic appearance lend support to periostitis as the etiology. However, as noted by Devas (1958), inflammation is a common finding in the region around a stress fracture.

To summarize, the available information on the medial tibial syndrome indicates that it most likely represents a stress reaction to the fascia, periosteum, and bone at this location of the leg, and not a compartment syndrome.

The treatment of this entity is widely disputed. It is obviously very resistant to the usual measures. In a prospective study of shin splints, Andrish et al. (1974) tried a variety of therapeutic measures. A majority of their patients exhibited the findings

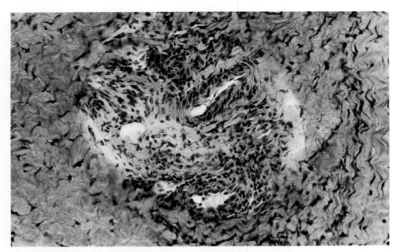

Figure 14–13 Photomicrograph (200 X) of fascia overlying deep posterior compartment of a patient with the medial tibial syndrome. This illustrates the inflammation and vasculitis noted in this entity.

of the medial tibial syndrome. Aspirin, phenylbutazone, heel-cord stretching, heel pads, and cast immobilization did not improve the overall results. Rest remained the treatment of choice for this particular entity. Jackson and Bailey (1975) reported no success with taping or arch supports, and also found that aspirin and local injection of steroids were not beneficial. They noted that a well cushioned shoe was of the most benefit subjectively. In a report of 20 patients, Clement (1974) recommends a two-phase approach. First, he employs rest including crutches and anti-inflammatory medication, and second, a graduated exercise program using isometric and isotonic exercises. The most divergent approach is that of Puranen (1974), who performed a deep posterior compartment fasciotomy in the 11 cases he reviewed, and reported satisfactory results in all patients.

We have taken an approach of treating these patients conservatively. The common denominator with all treatment modalities is rest, followed by resumption of sporting activities in a graduated fashion. Most cases will improve with time. Taping, arch supports, and alteration of shoe wear may help. In our experience, two patients have undergone deep posterior compartment fasciotomy. Both had bilateral symptomatology, but the surgery was performed on only the most involved side. Both individuals reported excellent improvement one year after the procedure, but neither returned for surgery on the contralateral side. If fasciotomy can benefit the more recalcitrant cases of this syndrome, a large, well controlled study will be necessary to prove this point. At this time we do not recommend surgical intervention for treatment of this entity.

Treatment of Chronic Compartment Syndrome

Once the diagnosis of a chronic exertional compartment syndrome of the leg has been established by history, examination, and pressure measurement, fasciotomy is usually required. However, in many cases, when the diagnosis and treatment is outlined to the patients, they will prefer to limit their running or alter their exercise program. With the chronic form there is not the urgent need for fasciotomy as with an acute compartment syndrome. Reneman (1975) noted ten patients who declined his recommended surgical decompression, and these were all symptomatic at 10 to 12 months' follow-up. Most patients in our experience who desire to maintain a given level of jogging or running will require fasciotomy.

Mavor (1956) was the first to treat a chronic compartment syndrome successfully with fasciotomy. Reneman (1975), who has the largest experience, uses a blind technique for decompression of the anterior compartment. He notes that this technique is not useful in the lateral compartment because of the location of the superficial peroneal nerve. Reneman uses a diathermic wire to burn through the fascia in order to minimize the skin incision.

We prefer a more direct and open approach. The necessary instruments for this procedure include right-angled retractors, a 12-inch Metzenbaum scissors, and/or a fasciotome*. For either anterior or lateral compartment involvement, both compartments are decompressed. The skin incision is in the midportion of the leg, halfway between the fibula and the anterior portion of the tibial crest (Mubarak and Owen, 1977). The usual length is 5 to 6 cm (Fig. 14–14). Muscle hernias are frequently noted in the lower third of the leg in the area overlying the anterior intermuscular septum. This is the site of emergence through the fascia of one or both sensory branches of the superficial peroneal nerve. If such a muscle hernia is present, the skin incision should be located over the hernia, so that one can explore the fascial defect and identify the superficial peroneal nerve (Fig. 14–6, see inset). Through this approach one can easily decompress both the anterior and lateral compartments. *Closure of this defect is never indicated because of the risk of precipitating an acute compartment syndrome* (Sirbu, 1944; Leach et al., 1967; Paton, 1968; Wolfort, 1973).

After making the skin incision, decompression of the anterior and lateral compartments is carried out as described in Chapter 10. The wound is closed with an intradermal running stitch, and a light dressing is applied. The patient is usually

---

*Made by Down Surgical Co., Toronto, Ont., Canada.

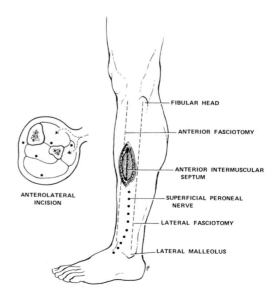

Figure 14–14 Anterolateral incision used to decompress the anterior and lateral compartments. When treating a chronic anterior compartment syndrome, the length of the skin incision may be considerably shorter (5 to 6 cm) than for an acute syndrome. (With permission from Mubarak, S. J., and Owen, C. A.: Double-incision fasciotomy of the leg for decompression of compartment syndromes. J. Bone Joint Surg. 59-A:184–187, 1977.)

ANTEROLATERAL INCISION

FIBULAR HEAD

ANTERIOR FASCIOTOMY

ANTERIOR INTERMUSCULAR SEPTUM

SUPERFICIAL PERONEAL NERVE

LATERAL FASCIOTOMY

LATERAL MALLEOLUS

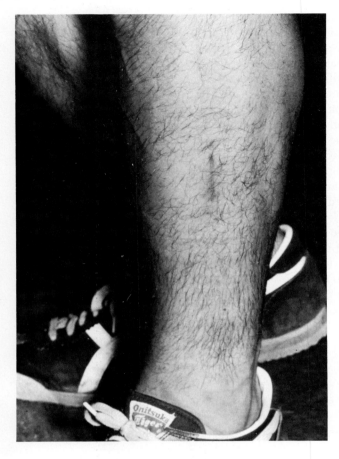

Figure 14–15 Well healed scar from anterolateral compartment fasciotomy performed one year previously on this marathon runner's left leg.

discharged the following day. Light exercises are begun within ten days and are gradually increased according to the patient's abilities (Fig. 14–15).

Follow-up studies on patients who have had surgical decompression demonstrate a more normal tissue pressure measurement during exercise. In Reneman's experience, the pressure at rest and after exercise does not completely return to normal limits. In the few whom we have had an opportunity to study following fasciotomy, tissue pressure measurements were essentially the same as those of normal runners (Table 14–3).

Table 14–3 ANTERIOR COMPARTMENTAL PRESSURE IN PATIENT WITH BILATERAL CHRONIC EXERTIONAL COMPARTMENT SYNDROMES: EFFECT OF FASCIOTOMY

	Resting Pressure Right/Left	Postexercise (5 Minutes) Right/Left
Prefasciotomy	15/16 mm Hg	28/28 mm Hg
Postfasciotomy (one year)	8/10 mm Hg	16/16 mm Hg

REFERENCES

Andrish, J. T., Bergfeld, J. A., and Walheim, J.: A prospective study on the management of shin splints. J. Bone Joint Surg. 56-A:1697–1700, 1974.

Anrep, G. V., Blalock, A., and Samaan, A.: The effect of muscular contraction upon blood flow in skeletal muscle. Proc. R. Soc. Lond. (Biol.) 114:223–245, 1934.

Ashton, H.: The effect of increased tissue pressure on blood flow. Clin. Orthop. 113:15–26, 1975.

Barcroft, H., and Millen, J. L. E.: The blood flow through muscle during sustained contraction. J. Physiol. 97:17–31, 1939.

Blandy, J. P., and Fuller, R.: March gangrene. J. Bone Joint Surg. 39-B:679–693, 1957.

Browne, S. G.: The anterior tibial compartment syndrome. Differential diagnosis in a Nigerian leprosarium. Br. J. Surg. 49:429, 1962.

Carter, A. B., Richards, R. L., and Zachary, R. B.: The anterior tibial syndrome. Lancet 2:928–934, 1949.

Clement, D. B.: Tibial stress syndrome in athletes. J. Sports Med. 2:81–85, 1974.

D'Ambrosia, R. D., Zelis, R. F., Chuinard, R. G., and Wilmore, J. Interstitial pressure measurements in the anterior and posterior compartments in athletes with shin splints. Am. J. Sports Med. 5:127–131, 1977.

Daniels, B. W., and Grennan, H. A.: Pretibial fever. J.A.M.A. 122:361–365, 1943.

Devas, M. B.: Stress fractures of the tibia in athletes or "shin splints." J. Bone Joint Surg. 40-B:227–239, 1958.

Ericksson, E., and Wallensten, R.: Can research into muscle morphology and muscle metabolism improve orthopaedic treatment? West Orthop. Assoc., Las Vegas, NV, Oct. 16, 1979.

Freedman, B. J.: Dr. Edward Wilson of the Antarctic; a biographical sketch, followed by an inquiry into the nature of his last illness. Proc. R. Soc. Med. 47:7–13, 1953.

French, E. B., and Price, W. H.: Anterior tibial pain. Br. Med. J. 2:1290–1296, 1962.

Garfin, S. R., Mubarak, S. J., and Owen, C. A.: Exertional anterolateral compartment syndrome. J. Bone Joint Surg. 59-A:404–405, 1977.

Grant, R. T.: Observations on the blood circulation in voluntary muscle in man. Clin. Sci. 3:157–173, 1938.

Griffiths, D. L.: The anterior tibial syndrome: a chronic form? J. Bone Joint Surg. 38-B:438–439, 1956.

Grunwald, A., and Silberman, Z.: Anterior tibial syndrome. J.A.M.A. 171:132–2210, 1959.

Hill, A. V.: The pressure developed in muscle during contraction. J. Physiol. 107:518–526, 1948.

Horn, C. E.: Acute ischaemia of the anterior tibial muscle and the long extensor muscles of the toes. J. Bone Joint Surg. 27-A:615–622, 1945.

Hughes, J. R.: Ischaemic necrosis of the anterior tibial muscles due to fatigue. J. Bone Joint Surg. 30-B:581–594, 1948.

Jackson, D. W., and Bailey, D.: Shin splints in the young athlete: a nonspecific diagnosis. Physician and Sports Med. 3:45–51, 1975.

Kennelly, B. M., and Blumberg, L.: Bilateral anterior tibial claudication. J.A.M.A. 203:487–491, 1968.

Kirby, N. G.: Exercise ischaemia in the fascial compartment of the soleus. J. Bone Joint Surg. 52-B:738–740, 1970.

Kjellmer, I.: An indirect method for estimating tissue pressure with special reference to tissue pressure in muscle during exercise. Acta Physiol. Scand. 62:31–40, 1964.

Kornstad, L.: Tibialis-anterior syndrome. Nord. Med. 53:694, 1955.

Kunkel, M. G., and Lynn, R. B.: The anterior tibial compartment syndrome. Can. J. Surg. 1:212–217, 1958.

Leach, R. E., Hammond, G., and Stryker, W. S.: Anterior tibial compartment syndrome: acute and chronic. J. Bone Joint Surg. 49-A:451–462, 1967.

Linge, B. van: Experimentele Spierhypertrofie bij de Rat. Van Garkum, Assen, 1959.

Mavor, G. E.: The anterior tibial syndrome. J. Bone Joint Surg. 38-B:513–517, 1956.

Mubarak, S. J., and Hargens, A. R.: Unpublished data, 1980.

Mubarak, S. J., Hargens, A. R., Owen, C. A., Akeson, W. H., and Garetto, L. P.: The wick catheter technique for measurement of intramuscular pressure; a new research and clinical tool. J. Bone Joint Surg. 58-A:1016–1020, 1976.

Mubarak, S. J., and Owen, C. A.: Double incision fasciotomy of the leg for decompression in compartment syndrome. J. Bone Joint Surg. 59-A:184–187, 1977.

Mubarak, S. J., Owen, C. A., Garfin, S. R., and Hargens, A. R.: Acute exertional superficial posterior compartment syndrome. Am. J. Sports Med. 6:287–290, 1978A.

Mubarak, S. J., Owen, C. A., Hargens, A. R., Garetto, L. P., and Akeson, W. H.: Acute compartment syndromes: diagnosis and treatment with the aid of the wick catheter. J. Bone Joint Surg. 60-A:1091–1095, 1978B.

Owen, C. A., Schmidt, D. A., Hargens, A. R., Garetto, L. P., Mubarak, S. J., and Akeson, W. H.: Intramuscular fluid pressure during isometric contraction. Unpublished data, 1981.

Paton, D. F.: The pathogenesis of anterior tibial syndrome. J. Bone Joint Surg. 50-B:383–385, 1968.

Pearson, C., Adams, R. D., and Denny-Brown, D.: Traumatic necrosis of pretibial muscles. N. Engl. J. Med. 231:213–217, 1948.

Puranen, J.: The medial tibial syndrome. Exercise ischaemia in the medial fascial compartment of the leg. J. Bone Joint Surg. 56-B:712–715, 1974.

Reid, R. L., and Travis, R. T.: Acute necrosis of the second interosseous compartment of the hand. J. Bone Joint Surg. 55-A:1095–1097, 1973.

Reneman, R. S.: The Anterior and the Lateral Compartment Syndrome of the Leg. Mouton Co., The Hague, 1968.

Reneman, R. S.: The anterior and the lateral compartment syndrome of the leg due to intensive use of muscles. Clin. Orthop. 113:69–80, 1975.

Schmidt, D. A., Owen, C. A., Hargens, A. R., Mubarak, S. J., and Akeson, W. H.: An assessment of isometric quadriceps exercises. Unpublished data, 1981.

Severin, E.: Unwandlung des Musculus tibialis anterior in Narbengewebe nach Uberanstrengung. Acta Chir. Scand. 89:426, 1944.

Sirbu, A. B., Murphy, M. J., and White, A. S.: Soft tissue complications of fractures of the leg. Calif. West. Med. 60:53–56, 1944.

Slocum, D. B.: The shin splint syndrome: medical aspects and differential diagnosis. Am. J. Surg. 114:875–881, 1967.

Snook, G. A.: Intermittent claudication in athletes. J. Sports Med. 3:71–75, 1975.

Tillotson, J. F., and Coventry, M. B.: Spontaneous ischemic necrosis of the anterior tibial muscle; report of a case. Proc. Mayo Clin. 25:223, 1950.

Tompkins, D. G.: Exercise myopathy of the extensor carpi ulnaris muscle. Report of a case. J. Bone Joint Surg. 59-A:407–408, 1977.

Vogt, P. R.: Ischemic muscular necrosis following marching. Oregon State Med. Soc., Sept. 4, 1943.

Wells, H. S., Youmans, J. B., and Miller, D. G., Jr.: Tissue pressure (intracutaneous, subcutaneous, and intramuscular) as related to venous pressure, capillary filtration, and other factors. J. Clin. Invest. 17:489–499, 1938.

Wolfort, F. G., Mogelvang, L. C., and Filtzer, H. S.: Anterior tibial compartment syndrome following muscle hernia repair. Arch. Surg. 106:97–99, 1973.

Wright, S.: Applied Physiology, 10th ed. Oxford University Press, London, 1961.

Index

Page number in *italics* indicates an illustration; page number followed by t indicates a table.